Handbook of
Cutaneous Melanoma

A Guide to Diagnosis and Treatment

T0100572

Handbook of Cutaneous Melanoma
A Guide to Diagnosis and Treatment

Dirk Schadendorf
University Hospital Essen
Department for Dermatology, Venereology and Allergology
Essen
Germany

Co-authors
Corinna Kochs
Elisabeth Livingstone
University Hospital Essen
Department for Dermatology
Essen
Germany

Springer Healthcare

Published by Springer Healthcare Ltd, 236 Gray's Inn Road, London, WC1X 8HB, UK.

www.springerhealthcare.com

British Library Cataloguing-in-Publication Data.

A catalogue record for this book is available from the British Library.

ISBN 978-1-908517-97-5

Although every effort has been made to ensure that drug doses and other information are presented accurately in this publication, the ultimate responsibility rests with the prescribing physician. Neither the publisher nor the authors can be held responsible for errors or for any consequences arising from the use of the information contained herein. Any product mentioned in this publication should be used in accordance with the prescribing information prepared by the manufacturers. No claims or endorsements are made for any drug or compound at present under clinical investigation.

Project editor: Alla Zarifyan and Tess Salazar
Designer: Joe Harvey
Artworker: Sissan Mollerfors
Production: Marina Maher
Printed in Great Britain by Latimer Trend

Contents

Biographies

Dirk Schadendorf, MD, is the Director of the Department of Dermatology at the University Hospital Essen, Germany. He attended medical school at the University Hospital, Hamburg, Germany, and has been licensed to practice medicine since 1986. In 1987, Professor Schadendorf went to Memorial Sloan-Kettering Cancer Center in New York, USA for 2 years, where he obtained a post-doctorate in tumor immunology. He spent 6 years at the Department of Dermatology at University Hospital Rudolf Virchow in Berlin, where he became board certified for dermatology and venereology and was Assistant Professor for Dermatology. Since 1995, Professor Schadendorf has also received board certification for allergology, quality management, medicamentous tumor therapy, and palliative medicine. After becoming a Heisenberg Scholar in 1997, he was made Associate Professor for Dermato-Oncology at Mannheim University Hospital, Medical Faculty of the University of Heidelberg, and Head of the Skin Cancer Unit at the German Cancer Research Center, Heidelberg, Germany. In his current role as the Director of the Department of Dermatology at University Hospital Essen, Professor Schadendorf is currently involved in 31 clinical studies. He is the current president of the German DeCOG (Dermatologic Cooperative Oncology Group) and chair-elect of the well-known EORTC Melanoma Group. He has a strong focus on translational research and has published more than 300 peer-reviewed papers.

Co-authors

Corinna Kochs, MD, is a resident at the Department of Dermatology, University Hospital Essen, Germany. She studied medicine at the Université Catholique de Louvain, Brussels, Belgium and at the Westfälische Wilhelms University, Münster, Germany. From 2011–2013, she was involved in the development of the German Melanoma Guideline 2013, published by the German Guideline Program in Oncology, where her main responsibilities were the project coordination and methodology. It is the first German Melanoma Guideline that contains evidence as well as GCP (good clinical practice)-based recommendations on diagnosis, therapy, and follow-up of cutaneous melanoma.

Elisabeth Livingstone, MD, is Attending Physician at the Department of Dermatology, University Hospital Essen, Germany. She studied medicine at Christian-Albrechts University, Kiel, Germany, where she also started her training in dermatology. Her main clinical and research activities are in the field of dermatooncology and cutaneous adverse events of new oncological substances. As sub-investigator, she has been involved in several phase II–III trials for melanoma and basal cell carcinoma.

Abbreviations

AJCC	American Joint Committee of Cancer
APC	antigen-presenting cell
CGH	comparative genomic hybridization
CT	computer tomography
CTLA-4	cytotoxic T-lymphocytic antigen-4
EMA	European Medicines Agency
FDA	US Food and Drug Administration
GM-CSF	granulocyte-macrophage colony-stimulating factor
HDAC	histone deacetylase
ICD-O-3	International Classification of Diseases for Oncology, 3rd edition
IFN	interferon
IHC	immunohistochemistry
IL-2	interleukin-2
LDH	lactate dehydrogenase
MHC	major histocompatibility complex
MRI	magnetic resonance imaging
NICE	National Institute for Health and Care Excellence
NOS	not otherwise specified
PD-1	programmed cell death-1
PET	positron emission tomography
RANKL	receptor activator of nuclear factor kappa-B ligand
SCREEN	Skin Cancer Research to Provide Evidence for Effectiveness of Screening in Northern Germany
SPECT	single photon emission computed tomography
T-VEC	talimogene laherparepvec
TA-99	tyrosinase-related protein antibody
TCR	T-cell receptor
TNF-α	tumor necrosis factor alpha
TNM	T, tumor, N, nodes, M, metastases
TRP-1	tyrosinase-related protein-1

UV	ultraviolet
wb	whole-body
WHO	World Health Organization

Introduction to cutaneous melanoma

Among all skin cancers, melanoma is the most aggressive, with increasing incidence worldwide and a high potential of metastatic spread. Survival rates in the metastatic stage are poor and therapy is limited. While many aspects of the etiology of melanoma are not yet clearly understood, several risk factors have been described and will be discussed later in this chapter [1–3]. In the past, therapy options remained limited and were only modestly effective in advanced disease. In recent years, research on melanoma has been progressing rapidly, and genetic and immuno-logic factors associated with melanoma development and progression have been identified, offering avenues for new therapeutic strategies, including immunomodulating and targeted agents.

"Malignant melanoma" and "melanoma" are synonymous terms; the latter will be used in this book.

Epidemiology: incidence and mortality

The incidence of cutaneous melanoma has been increasing worldwide in white populations for several decades, especially in young adults and women, making melanoma one of the most rapidly increasing cancers in white populations [1,4,5]. The incidence and mortality of melanoma compared to other common cancers is shown in Figure 1.1 [6].

The highest incidence rates have been reported in Australia and New Zealand [7], and approximately 132,000 cases of melanoma are reported globally each year [8]. For 2013, it is estimated that there will

D. Schadendorf et al., *Handbook of Cutaneous Melanoma*,
DOI· 10.1007/978-1-908517-98-2_1, © Springer Healthcare 2013

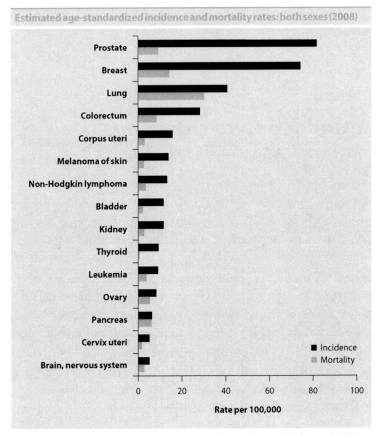

Figure 1.1 Estimated age-standardized incidence and mortality rates: both sexes (2008).
Reproduced with permission from Ferlay J, Shin HR, Bray F, Forman D, Mathers C and Parkin DM.
GLOBOCAN 2008, Cancer Incidence and Mortality Worldwide: IARC CancerBase No. 10 [Internet].
Lyon, France: International Agency for Research on Cancer; 2010 [6].

be 76,690 new melanoma cases with 9480 deaths [4]. Additionally, approximately 61,300 melanomas in situ will be newly diagnosed in 2013 [4].

As melanoma is generally detected at an early invasive stage (T1), the 5-year survival rate is above 90% for women and 87% for men in Western Europe and North America [9]. However, survival from melanoma is poorer in older patients and when it is diagnosed at a later stage [10]. Once melanoma has spread and metastases have developed, the overall survival rate is dismal: while the 5-year survival rate in patients without metastases is about 98%, it is only about 15% in patients with distant metastatic disease [4].

Pathogenesis

Melanoma is a neoplasm that originates from melanocytes, a specialized cell type located in the epidermis that is responsible for the production of the melanin pigments (Figure 1.2). Two types of melanin determine phenotypic features: while the reddish-yellow eumelanin is predominant

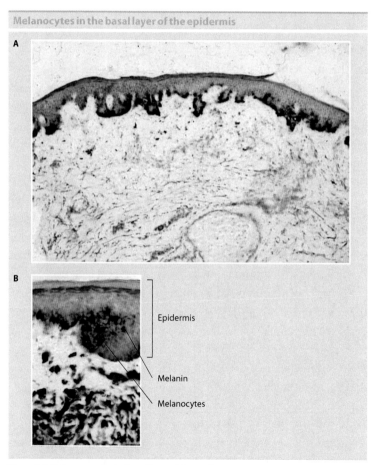

Figure 1.2 Melanocytes in the basal layer of the epidermis. Immunohistological staining with tyrosinase-related protein-1 (TRP-1)-specific antibody, TA-99 antibody. (A) size 10x; (B) size 40x.

in light-complexioned subjects (grey, blue, or green eyes; blond or red hair; freckles), the dark pheomelanin is found in dark-complexioned subjects (brown eyes; dark hair) [11,12].

Melanoma can develop on pre-existing moles such as a congenital, acquired, or atypical nevus, but more than half of all melanomas develop de novo [9,13]. Several risk factors associated with the development of melanoma have been identified and will be discussed in the next section. Over the last decade, various immunologic processes and genetic alterations associated with the pathogenesis of melanoma have been identified and will be discussed in this chapter as well.

Risk factors

Environmental risk factors

Ultraviolet (UV) radiation, one major risk factor for melanoma development, was described in 1991 by the consensus panel Sunlight, Ultraviolet Radiation, and the Skin [14]. Later studies have confirmed that UV radiation is the major environmental risk factor and that people who are intermittently exposed have a higher risk of developing melanoma [2].

A history of sunburn was also identified as an important risk factor, and the risk is slightly higher for sunburns experienced in childhood compared with those in adulthood [2,7]. The association between sunburns and melanoma was greater in higher altitudes, although studies carried out in lower altitudes were also able to demonstrate an association between sunburns and melanoma [2].

One explanation for why UV radiation is so damaging is that it leads to cell and DNA damage and thus increases the risk of mutation [15,16]. People with signs of actinic damage of the skin, such as solar lentigo, elastosis, actinic keratosis, and nonmelanocytic cutaneous tumors (eg, squamous cell carcinoma and/or basal cell carcinoma), are at higher risk of developing melanoma [3].

Acquired and genetic risk factors

The number of congenital or acquired common and atypical nevi is a very important independent risk factor for the occurrence of melanoma [1,17]. The term "atypical nevi" is frequently used for nevi that are clinically suspected of underlying dysplasia [1]. It was shown that people with at least five atypical nevi have a sixfold higher risk of developing melanoma than people without atypical nevi [1]. Having numerous moles is possibly related to a genetic predisposition for melanoma development. Increased UV radiation exposure may not only lead to the development of multiple moles but also to an increased risk of melanoma transformation [1,17].

The Fitzpatrick standard classification distinguishes different skin types according to the color of the skin and eyes and the patients' burning or tanning response to sunlight exposure (Table 1.1) [18,19]. Photosensitivity is increased in people with a light complexion and freckles compared to people with a dark skin type, and an association of photosensitivity with melanoma is assumed [3]. It should also be noted that constitutional UV sensitivity is not only a risk factor for the development of melanoma, but also for nonmelanoma skin cancers, such as squamous cell carcinoma and/or basal cell carcinoma in whites [3,7].

Personal history of a previous melanoma and a positive family history of melanoma, usually defined as the diagnosis of melanoma in one or more affected first-degree relatives, is associated with a higher risk for the development of melanomas [3,15,20]. More information on familial melanoma can be found through the Melanoma Genetics Consortium [21].

Fitzpatrick skin type according to phenotype and sun exposure

Skin type (Fitzpatrick standard classification)	Phenotype	Response to sun exposure
I	White skin, very fair; freckles; red or blonde hair; blue eyes	Always burns, never tans
II	White skin; fair or blonde hair; blue, hazel, or green eyes	Usually burns, tans with difficulty
III	White or olive skin tone; fair with any eye or hair color	Sometimes mild burn, gradually tans
IV	Brown skin (typical Mediterranean Caucasian skin)	Rarely burns, tans with ease
V	Dark brown skin (Middle-Eastern skin types)	Very rarely burns, tans easily
VI	Black skin	Never burns, tans very easily

Table 1.1 Fitzpatrick skin type according to phenotype and sun exposure. Adapted from Freedberg et al [18] and the International Classification of Diseases for Oncology [19].

Take-home message

Risk factors for melanoma:

- Sunlight, UV radiation
- Number of nevi
- Phenotype (ligh complexion, freckled) and increased sun sensitivity
- Personal history of melanoma
- Family history of melanoma

Immunologic factors

Two components of the immune system, the humoral and the cell-mediated immune response, are considered of utmost importance for antitumor immunity [22]. One of the most important mechanisms is the elimination of tumor cells by cytotoxic CD8+ T lymphocytes. However, cancer cells are able to modify immunologic pathways and interactions to their own advantage and survival [22]. Mechanisms assumed to lead to tumor resistance include downregulated or disabled antigen presentation, immunologic barriers within the tumor microenvironment, negative regulatory pathways targeting T-cells, or T-cell dysfunction [23,24].

For example, one critical inhibitory signal is mediated by the interaction between cytotoxic T lymphocyte antigen-4 (CTLA-4) on T cells and its ligands (B7–1 and B7–2) on antigen-presenting cells (Figure 1.3) [25,26]. CTLA–4 is not strongly expressed on naive T cells but becomes rapidly induced after T-cell activation: the mechanism that prevents undesired autoimmunity and establishes tolerance to self-antigens by downregulating T-cell activation via a homeostatic feedback loop. However, this downregulatory mechanism can be modified in melanoma to disrupt the normal T-cell function, leading to a decreased antitumor response.

The expanding knowledge of immunologic processes in melanoma has resulted in the development and application of different immunomodulating therapy approaches (eg, interferon, vaccines) in order to support the body's tumor defense mechanisms. In recent years, selective antibodies, such as the CTLA-4 antibody ipilimumab, were explored as effective therapy strategies (see Chapter 5).

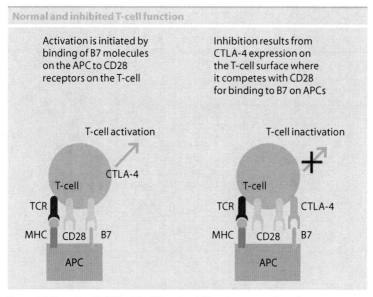

Figure 1.3 Normal and inhibited T-cell function. APC, antigen-presenting cell; CTLA-4, cytotoxic T lymphocyte antigen-4; TCR, T-cell receptor; MHC, major histocompatibility complex. Reproduced with permission from Tarhini et al [26].

Signaling aberrations associated with melanoma development

Research has led to further advances in the molecular understanding of the pathogenesis of melanoma. A variety of inherited and acquired genetic factors were identified in melanocytes as potential contributing factors in the development of melanoma either by activation of certain oncogenes or by inactivation of specific tumor suppressor genes.

One major finding is the upregulation of the BRAF-MEK-ERK transduction pathway. It is a cascade of several proteins that transmit a signal received from a receptor on the surface of the melanocyte to the DNA in the nucleolus. This cascade influences the regulation of a variety of cellular processes, including growth, survival, and migration [11]. Mutations in several genes (eg, BRAF, NRAS, c-KIT) lead to an activation of this pathway and thus oncogenesis (Figure 1.4) [27,28].

About half of all melanomas harbor an oncogenic mutation in the BRAF gene, which usually results in a single amino acid change at codon

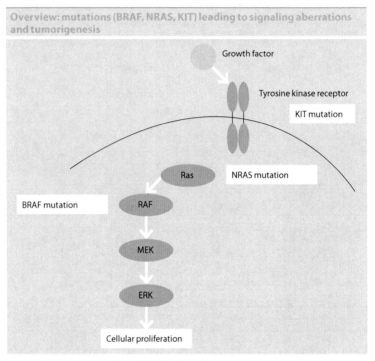

Overview: mutations (BRAF, NRAS, KIT) leading to signaling aberrations and tumorigenesis

Growth factor

Tyrosine kinase receptor

KIT mutation

Ras

NRAS mutation

BRAF mutation

RAF

MEK

ERK

Cellular proliferation

Figure 1.4 Overview: mutations (BRAF, NRAS, KIT) leading to signaling aberrations and tumorigenesis.

600 (BRAF^{V600E}) [18]. As a result of this BRAF mutation, cells receive continuous growth signals, leading to clonal expansion and tumor progression [11,27]. Mutations in NRAS or c-KIT are primarily found in acral and mucosal melanomas (which account for about 10–15% of all melanomas) [29].

The discovery of mutated oncogenic kinases offers a therapeutic approach through targeted therapies that selectively bind to tyrosine kinases and thus inhibit the signal transduction. Among these targeted drugs are selective BRAF inhibitors, such as vemurafenib and dabrafenib (both potent inhibitors of mutated BRAF), and MEK-inhibitors, such as trametinib. Vemurafenib was first approved by the US Food and Drug Administration (FDA) in 2011 for the treatment of advanced melanoma and dabrafenib was approved in May 2013; MEK-inhibitor trametinib was approved in the USA in May 2013 [26] (see Chapters 5 and 6).

Furthermore, families with a high susceptibility to melanoma have been observed and studied to elucidate potential pathways involved in pathogenesis [11,15]. Analyses showed a variety of distinct mutations that occur most commonly and with a high penetrance in genes, such as CDKN2A and CDK4, that are involved in cell cycle arrest and melanocyte senescence. Somatic mutations in these genes cause loss of function, which can result in melanoma progression [11].

Other mutations with low penetrance were found in the general population in or near genes that play a major role in hair and skin pigmentation (eg, MC1R, ASIP, TYR, TYRP1). These mutations in combination with external environmental factors (eg, sun exposure) may potentially influence melanoma development; however, this has not yet been clarified with certainty [11].

It is important to note that the development and progression of melanoma has a complicated etiology that is still somewhat elusive. It involves not only single-gene mutations but a whole complex of different inherited and acquired genetic factors as well as the mutagenic impact of UV radiation and other environmental factors [11,30].

Take-home message

UV radiation and subsequent DNA damage are major contributing factors for melanoma development. However, the pathogenesis of melanoma is complex and not yet fully elucidated. Defined molecular driver mutations have been identified in a significant subset of patients.

Prevention and screening

Prevention (primary prevention)

Sun exposure is a major causative factor in the development of melanoma. Therefore, efforts to educate the general public about the risks of sun exposure and to support sun avoidance (particularly important in childhood) have been made. In Australia, behavioral changes have been observed (eg, wearing sun-protective clothing on the school playground, less reported tanning and sunburns), but such campaigns were not equally successful in other countries, and sun exposure and tanning are still popular [7]. Although there is currently a lack of evidence that primary prevention leads to a decrease in overall melanoma-specific survival, it offers the potential to positively influence mortality in the long term [7].

Whether sunscreen protects against cutaneous melanoma has not been fully proven. However, sunscreen has been shown to reduce the risk of squamous cell carcinoma, so its use is advisable as well. People need to be informed that the application of sunscreen should not be used to increase the time spent in the sun and that sensible sun-protective behavior is mandatory (eg, avoidance of sun exposure, especially between 11 AM and 3 PM) [31]. In addition to sunscreen, the use of sun-protective clothing (eg, hats, sunglasses) is recommended, as that can minimize the amount of solar UV radiation exposure [11,30].

Screening (secondary prevention)

Screening programs can initially lead to a greater incidence of melanoma due to increased detection, but may eventually reduce tumor burden and thus decrease mortality, as was shown in Germany during and after SCREEN (Skin Cancer Research to Provide Evidence for Effectiveness of Screening in Northern Germany), the world's largest screening project [32]. The reason for both is that melanoma is detected at an earlier stage and that excision of thin or in situ melanoma offers the possibility of mortality reduction in the short term [7,31]. Even if screening programs are currently not implemented worldwide, there is hope that melanoma deaths can be reduced through prevention and screening [7,10].

Take-home message
Screening and prevention may help to reduce the incidence and mortality rate of skin cancer.

References

1   Gandini S, Sera F, Cattaruzza MS, et al. Meta-analysis of risk factors for cutaneous melanoma: I. Common and atypical naevi. *Eur J Cancer*. 2005;41:28-44.
2   Gandini S, Sera F, Cattaruzza MS, et al. Meta-analysis of risk factors for cutaneous melanoma: II. Sun exposure. *Eur J Cancer*. 2005;41:45-60.
3   Gandini S, Sera F, Cattaruzza MS, et al. Meta-analysis of risk factors for cutaneous melanoma: III. Family history, actinic damage and phenotypic factors. *Eur J Cancer*. 2005;41:2040-2059.
4   Cancer Facts & Figures 2010. American Cancer Society. www.cancer.org/downloads/STT/ Cancer_Facts_and_Figures_2010.pdf. Accessed June 20, 2013.

5 Reed KB, Brewer JD, Lohse CM, Bringe KE, Pruitt CN, Gibson LE. Increasing incidence of melanoma among young adults: an epidemiological study in Olmsted County, Minnesota. *Mayo Clin Proc*. 2012;87:328-334.

6 GLOBOCAN 2008 (IARC) Section of Cancer Information. FAST STATS. World. globocan.iarc.fr/factsheets/populations/factsheet.asp?uno=900. Accessed June 20, 2013.

7 Giblin AV, Thomas JM. Incidence, mortality and survival in cutaneous melanoma. *J Plast Reconstr Aesthet Surg*. 2007;60:32-40.

8 Ultraviolet radiation and the INTERSUN Programme. World Health Organization. www.who.int/uv/faq/skincancer/en/index1.html. Accessed June 20, 2013.

9 Kaatsch P, Spix C, Katalinic A, Hentschel S. Malignes Melanom der Haut. In: *Krebs in Deutschland 2007/2008*. Berlin, Germany: Robert Koch-Institut; 2012.

10 Pollack LA, Li J, Berkowitz Z, et al. Melanoma survival in the United States, 1992 to 2005. *J Am Acad Dermatol*. 2011;65(5 suppl 1): S78.e.1-S78.e.10.

11 Meyle KD, Guldberg P. Genetic risk factors for melanoma. *Hum Genet*. 2009;126:499-510.

12 Sturm RA. Molecular genetics of human pigmentation diversity. *Hum Mol Genet*. 2009;18:R9-R17.

13 Clark WH Jr, From L, Bernardino EA, Mihm MC. The histogenesis and biologic behavior of primary human malignant melanomas of the skin. *Cancer Res*. 1969;29:705-727.

14 National Institutes of Health summary of the Consensus Development Conference on Sunlight, Ultraviolet Radiation, and the Skin. Bethesda, Maryland, May 8-10, 1989. Consensus Development Panel. *J Am Acad Dermatol*. 1991;24:608-612.

15 Horn S, Figl A, Rachakonda PS, et al. TERT promoter mutations in familial and sporadic melanoma. *Science*. 2013;339:959-961.

16 Gilchrest BA, Eller MS, Geller AC, Yaar M. The pathogenesis of melanoma induced by ultraviolet radiation. *N Engl J Med*. 1999;340:1341-1348.

17 Stierner U, Augustsson A, Rosdahl I, Suurküla M. Regional distribution of common and dysplastic naevi in relation to melanoma site and sun exposure. A case-control study. *Melanoma Res*. 1992;1:367-375.

18 Freedberg IM, Eisen AZ, Wolff K, Austen KF, Goldsmith LA, Katz SI, eds. *Fitzpatrick´s Dermatology in General Medicine*. 5th edn. New York, NY: McGraw-Hill; 1999.

19 International Classification of Diseases for Oncology. 3rd edn (ICD-O-3). Geneva, Switzerland: World Health Organization; 2000.

20 Rhodes AR, Weinstock MA, Fitzpatrick TB, Mihm MC, Sober AJ. Risk factors for cutaneous melanoma. A practical method of recognizing predisposed individuals. *JAMA*. 1987;258:3146-3154.

21 The Melanoma Genetics Consortium. www.genomel.org. Accessed June 20, 2013.

22 de Visser KE, Eichten A, Coussens LM. Paradoxical roles of the immune system during cancer development. *Nat Rev Cancer*. 2006;6:24-37.

23 Gajewski TF. Failure at the effector phase: immune barriers at the level of the melanoma tumor microenvironment. *Clin Cancer Res*. 2007;13:5256-5261.

24 Drake CG, Jaffee E, Pardoll DM. Mechanisms of immune evasion by tumors. *Adv Immunol*. 2006;90:51-81.

25 Ji Z, Flaherty KT, Tsao H. Targeting the RAS pathway in melanoma. *Trends Mol Med*. 2012;18:27-35.

26 Tarhini A, Lo E, Minor DR. Releasing the brake on the immune system: ipilimumab in melanoma and other tumors. *Cancer Biother Radiopharm*. 2010;25:601-613.

27 Sullivan RJ, Flaherty KT. BRAF in melanoma: pathogenesis, diagnosis, inhibition, and resistance. *J Skin Cancer*. 2011;2011:423239.

28 Ji Z, Flaherty KT, Tsao H. Targeting the RAS pathway in melanoma. *Trends Mol Med*. 2012;18:27-35.

29 Glud M, Gniadecki R. MicroRNAs in the pathogenesis of malignant melanoma. *J Eur Acad Dermatol Venereol*. 2013;27:142-150.

30 Hodis E, Watson IR, Kryukov GV, et al. A landscape of driver mutations in melanoma. *Cell*. 2012;150:251-263.

31 Planta MB. Sunscreen and melanoma: is our prevention message correct? *J Am Board Fam Med*. 2011;24:735-739.

32 Breitbart EW, Waldmann A, Nolte S, et al. Systematic skin cancer screening in Northern Germany. *J Am Acad Dermatol*. 2012;66:201-211.

Chapter 2

Clinical features and classification

Subtypes of melanoma

Clinicopathologic subtypes

Clark et al [1] were the first to divide melanoma into subtypes depending on clinical and histologic features, criteria that were later used by other researchers [2]. The majority of all melanomas fall into the following four subtypes (the World Health Organization [WHO] classification of melanoma) (Table 2.1) [1–5]:

- Superficial spreading
- Nodular
- Lentigo maligna
- Acral lentiginous

Precursor lesions with no penetration of the basal membrane but with a high risk of transforming into melanoma are called "melanoma in situ" or "lentigo maligna." The superficial cells of the primary lesion, either intraepidermal or just below the basal membrane, determine the classification of melanoma. Lesions without pigment are classified as "amelanotic" [1]. Nodular and acral lentiginous melanomas have the poorest 5-year survival rates among all histological subtypes (69.4% and 81.2%, respectively), mainly because of their higher tumor thickness at the time of diagnosis [6].

The WHO classification includes further subtypes listed in Table 2.2 [7]. One rare melanoma subtype is the desmoplastic melanoma that is often amelanotic and can be difficult to diagnose. Histopathologically, perineural invasion is an atypical feature of this desmoplastic melanoma

D. Schadendorf et al., *Handbook of Cutaneous Melanoma*, DOI: 10.1007/978-1-908517-98-2_2, © Springer Healthcare 2013

Overview of the four major melanoma subtypes

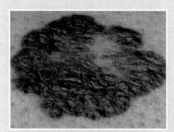

Superficial spreading melanoma is the most common subtype [3]. It frequently presents with diffused borders, a combination of several colors such as brown, black, red, white, or others, and an irregular and elevated surface. It is characterized by laterally spreading melanocytes within the epidermis, making the assessment of the lateral extent of the melanoma difficult [1,2].

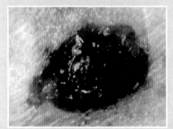

Nodular melanoma is another common subtype. In contrast to the superficial spreading melanoma, the nodular melanoma presents with a relatively sharp border as the melanocytes extend vertically rather than horizontally [1,2].

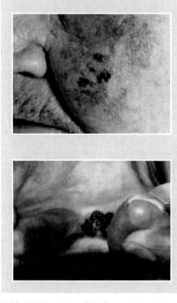

Lentigo maligna or **Lentigo maligna melanoma** usually develops on sun-damaged skin (eg, on the head and neck area of elderly patients). Lentigo maligna is a melanoma in situ and a precursor lesion for the lentigo maligna melanoma. Distinction from "actinic melanocytosis" (increased intraepidermal melanocytes secondary to chronic sun exposure) can be difficult [2]. Contrary to the melanoma in situ, lentigo maligna melanoma invades the dermis.

Acral lentiginous melanoma is rare in the white population but appears in higher proportions in other races (in particular in Blacks, Asians, and Pacific Islanders) [4]. It is found on acral regions, such as the palms of the hands, the soles of the feet, within nail beds, or under nail plates [2,5]. Diagnosis is often delayed due to the hidden location or because it can be mistaken for an ulcer or a plantar wart with hemorrhage.

Table 2.1 Overview of the four major melanoma subtypes. Adapted from Clark et al [1], Smoller et al [2], Kaatsch et al [3], Bradford et al [4], and Glud et al [5].

Melanoma subtypes according to the WHO classification	
Melanoma subtypes	**ICD-O-3 codes**
Malignant melanoma – major subtypes	**M8720/3**
Superficial spreading melanoma	M8743/3
Nodular melanoma	M8721/3
Lentigo maligna melanoma	M8742/3
Acral lentiginous melanoma	M8744/3
Other	
Desmoplastic melanoma	M8745/3
Melanoma arising from a blue nevus	M8780/3
Melanoma arising in a giant congenital nevus	M8761/3
Melanoma in childhood	
Naevoid melanoma	M8720/3
Melanoma, NOS	

Table 2.2 Melanoma subtypes according to the WHO classification. ICD-O-3, International Classification of Diseases for Oncology, 3rd edition; NOS, not otherwise specified; WHO, World Health Organization. Adapted from the World Health Organization [7].

that leads to higher rates of local relapses. In some cases (<10%) desmoplastic melanomas also display components of a nondesmoplastic melanoma (so-called mixed desmoplastic melanoma in contrast to pure desmoplastic melanoma) [8].

Take-home message

Different melanoma subtypes can be distinguished. The four major subtypes (according to the WHO classification and on the basis of clinical and histological features) are:

- Superficial spreading melanoma
- Nodular melanoma
- Lentigo maligna melanoma
- Acral lentiginous melanoma

Genetic alterations in melanoma subtypes

Cutaneous melanoma is a heterogeneous disease with different clinico-pathologic subtypes. However, in clinical practice, a substantial number of melanomas do not fit into the classic subtypes. More recently, mutation analyses showed that melanomas can also be classified according to distinct genetic alterations in different pathways, which also helps to better understand why melanomas develop and explains some of the biologic features [9]. These findings served as the foundation for the development of the first targeted therapies in melanoma. The different subtypes are summarized in Table 2.3 [10].

Another approach for a genetic classification of melanomas, proposed by Bastian et al, relates to their preferential body site of occurrence and exposure to ultraviolet (UV) radiation [11]. Mutations in BRAF and chromosomal losses (chromosome 10) were shown to occur significantly more often in melanoma of intermittently sun-exposed skin, while mutations in NRAS were mostly found in melanoma in sun-protected areas (eg, acral lentiginous melanoma) [11]. The role of sun exposure or sun damage to the skin in the development of acral lentiginous melanoma is assumed to be of lesser importance [9].

Principal melanoma molecular subtypes				
Detailed subtypes	Pathway(s)	Key gene/ biomarker(s)	Diagnostic technologies	Potentially relevant therapeutics
1.1	MAPK	BRAF	Targeted sequencing	BRAF inhibitors, MEK inhibitors, Hsp90 inhibitors
1.2		BRAF/PTEN	Targeted sequencing and IHC	(BRAF inhibitors) and (PI3K, AKT, or mTOR inhibitors)
1.3		BRAF/AKT	Targeted sequencing and copy number	(BRAF inhibitors) and (AKT or mTOR inhibitors)
1.4		BRAF/CDK4	Targeted sequencing and copy number/CGH	BRAF inhibitors and CDK inhibitors
2.1	c-KIT	c-KIT	Targeted sequencing	Imatinib and other c-KIT inhibitors
3.1	GNAQ, GNA11	GNAQ	Targeted sequencing	MEK inhibitors
3.2		GNA11	Targeted sequencing	MEK inhibitors
4.1	NRAS	NRAS	Targeted sequencing	MEK and PI3K inhibitors and farnesyltransferase inhibitors
5.1	MITF	MITF	Copy number	HDAC inhibitors

Table 2.3 Principal melanoma molecular subtypes. CGH, comparative genomic hybridization; HDAC, histone deacetylase; IHC, immunohistochemistry. Adapted from Vidwans et al [10].

Despite the many investigations in this field and a rapidly growing knowledge base, classification according to specific mutational profiles is not yet validated. Further investigations are required for validation and refinement, and to possibly identify additional factors.

Take-home message

Different key molecular pathways are involved in melanoma disease onset and progression. Classification of different melanoma subtypes on the basis of genetic factors (in contrast to traditional clinical pathologic subtypes) has been proposed but requires validation.

American Joint Committee on Cancer staging and classification

Melanoma staging is based on the American Joint Committee on Cancer (AJCC) TNM classification system (T=tumor, N=nodes, M=metastases), which was developed in 2009 on the basis of long-term follow-up data of more than 38,000 patients (Table 2.4) [12]. The anatomic stage groupings for cutaneous melanoma are based on the TNM staging (Table 2.5) [12]. Compared to previous classification systems (eg, AJCC 2002) [13], mitotic rate has been added as a prognostic factor in low-risk melanoma, replacing the level of invasion (Clark level). According to the TNM classification, the Clark level is only used for the subdivision between T1a and T1b if the mitotic rate was not assessed. Sentinel node biopsy is required for the correct N-classification [12].

Patients with melanoma of unknown primary should be allocated to stage III (in case of skin and/or lymph node metastases) or IV disease, depending on the site(s) of metastases.

Prognostic factors and course of disease

Melanoma is the most serious form of skin cancer because it metastasizes so readily. The clinical course of cutaneous melanoma can be severe and depends on several prognostic factors. The Individualized Melanoma Patient Outcome Prediction Tool website (www.melanomaprognosis.org), found at the AJCC Melanoma Database, allows the provider to enter all

Classification	Thickness (mm)	Ulceration status/Mitoses
Tis	Not applicable	Not applicable
T1	≤1.00	a: without ulceration and mitosis <1/mm²
		b: with ulceration or mitoses ≥1/mm²
T2	1.01–2.00	a: without ulceration
		b: with ulceration
T3	2.01–4.00	a: without ulceration
		b: with ulceration
T4	>4.00	a: without ulceration
		b: with ulceration
Classification (N)	**Number of metastatic nodes**	**Nodal metastatic burden**
N0	0	Not applicable
N1	1	a: micrometastasis*
		b: macrometastases†
N2	2–3	a: micrometastasis*
		b: macrometastases†
		c: in-transit metastases/satellites without metastatic lymph nodes
N3	4+ metastatic lymph nodes, or matted lymph nodes, or in-transit metastases/satellites with metastatic lymph nodes	
Classification (M)	**Site**	**Serum LDH**
M0	No distant metastases	Not applicable
M1a	Distant skin, subcutaneous, or nodal metastases	Normal
M1b	Lung metastases	Normal
M1c	All other visceral metastases	Normal
	Any distant metastases	Elevated

Table 2.4 AJCC TNM staging categories for cutaneous melanoma (2009). *Micrometastases are diagnosed after sentinel lymph node biopsy. †Macrometastases are defined as clinically detectable nodal metastases confirmed pathologically. AJCC, American Joint Committee of Cancer; LDH, lactate dehydrogenase; M, metastases; N, nodes; T, tumor. Reproduced with permission from Balch et al [12].

of these factors to calculate the 5- and 10-year survival probability at the time of primary diagnosis [14].

	Clinical staging*				**Pathologic staging†**		
	T	**N**	**M**		**T**	**N**	**M**
0	Tis	N0	M0	0	Tis	N0	M0
IA	T1a	N0	M0	IA	T1a	N0	M0
IB	T1b	N0	M0	IB	T1b	N0	M0
	T2a	N0	M0		T2a	N0	M0
IIA	T2b	N0	M0	IIA	T2b	N0	M0
	T3a	N0	M0		T3a	N0	M0
IIB	T3b	N0	M0	IIB	T3b	N0	M0
	T4a	N0	M0		T4a	N0	M0
IIC	T4b	N0	M0	IIC	T4b	N0	M0
III	Any T	N> N0	M0	IIIA	T1-4a	N1a	M0
					T1-4a	N2a	M0
				IIIB	T1-4b	N1a	M0
					T1-4b	N2a	M0
					T1-4a	N1b	M0
					T1-4a	N2b	M0
					T1-4a	N2c	M0
				IIIC	T1-4b	N1b	M0
					T1-4b	N2b	M0
					T1-4b	N2c	M0
					Any T	N3	M0
IV		Any N		IV	Any T	Any N	M1

Table 2.5 Anatomic staging groups for cutaneous melanoma. *Clinical staging includes microstaging of the primary melanoma and clinical/radiologic evaluation for metastases. By convention, it should be used after complete excision of the primary melanoma with clinical assessment for regional and distant metastases. †Pathologic staging includes microstaging of the primary melanoma and pathologic information about the regional lymph nodes after partial (ie, sentinel node biopsy) or complete lymphadenectomy. Pathologic stage 0 or stage IA patients are the exception as they do not require pathologic evaluation of their lymph nodes. M, metastases; N, nodes; T, tumor. Reproduced with permission from Balch et al [12].

Prognostic factors

The following risk factors [12] are described and incorporated into the 2009 AJCC classification system:

- **Tumor thickness** is the most important prognostic factor. In patients with melanomas with tumor thickness ≤1.00 mm, the 10-year survival rate was shown to be about 92%, compared with 80% in patients with melanomas of 1.01–2.00-mm thickness, 63% in patients with melanomas of 2.01–4.00-mm thickness, and 50% in patients with melanomas of >4.00-mm thickness [12].

- **Ulceration** has an important influence on survival. Patients with an ulcerated T4 melanoma (pT4b) have a 5-year survival rate of 53%, while the survival rate for patients with a nonulcerated T4 primary (pT4a) ranges around 71% [12].

- The **mitotic rate** is a marker for the proliferation of the primary melanoma. A highly significant correlation between increasing mitotic rate and declining survival rates was demonstrated. The most significant correlation with survival was identified at a threshold of at least $1/mm^2$. Survival rates of patients with an ulcerated primary or elevated mitotic rate are lower than those of patients with a nonulcerated melanoma of equivalent T-category [12].

- **Nodular involvement**-related survival rates differ due to heterogeneity. Tumor burden at the time of staging (microscopic versus macroscopic) was shown to be a further prognostic factor. Five-year survival rates within stage III were 78%, 59%, and 40% for patients with stage IIIA, IIIB, and IIIC melanoma, respectively (Figure 2.1) [12].

- Prognosis is worse in patients with distant metastases. **Lactate dehydrogenase** (LDH) is a highly significant predictor of survival or outcome in stage IV patients, independent of other factors (Figure 2.2) [12]. When elevated LDH levels are found, patients are classified as M1c regardless of the location of distant metastases. One-year survival rates are approximately 62% (M1a), 53% (M1b), and 33% (M1c), respectively. Survival rates after 10 years range between 5% and 20% [12].

Other clinical factors of prognostic importance for survival include gender (males with poorer prognoses than females), increasing patient age, and location of the primary tumor (trunk and head sites have poorer prognosis than extremities) [13,15,16]; however, these factors are not included in the 2009 AJCC classification system [12,13].

> *Take-home message*
>
> Staging of patients is based on the 2009 AJCC classification, a TNM staging system that accounts for important prognostic factors:
>
> - Tumor thickness
> - Ulceration
> - Mitotic rate (in melanoma with a tumor thickness <1 mm)
> - Nodular involvement
> - LDH levels (in stage IV)
> - Additional known prognostic factors such as gender, age, and localization of the primary melanoma

Rate of growth

Early detection of melanoma before metastatic spread is of great importance. Diagnostic delay can have severe consequences, particularly in cases of rapidly growing melanomas. The spectrum of the growth rate varies widely, and growth rates from 0.03 mm/month in a slowly growing lentigo maligna melanoma and up to 1.48 mm/month in a rapidly growing nodular melanoma have been reported [17].

The assessment of clinical factors related to rapidly growing melanomas demonstrated the following associated factors [17]:

- Tumor thickness
- Mitotic rate
- Male sex
- Older age (≥70 years)
- Fewer melanocytic nevi and freckles (n<50)
- Atypical clinical features (eg, asymmetry, elevation, amelanosis, border irregularity, presence of symptoms)

> *Take-home message*
>
> When melanoma is suspected, rapid diagnosis and treatment are mandatory.

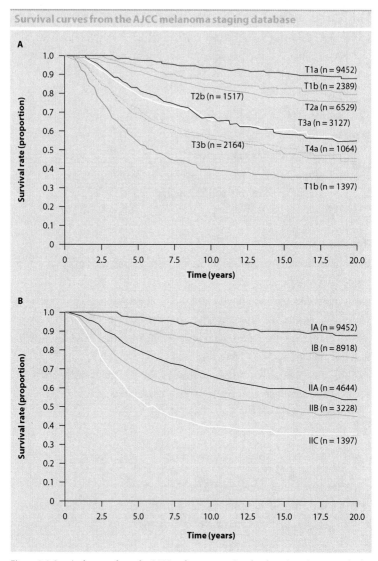

Figure 2.1 Survival curves from the AJCC melanoma staging database (continues overleaf).

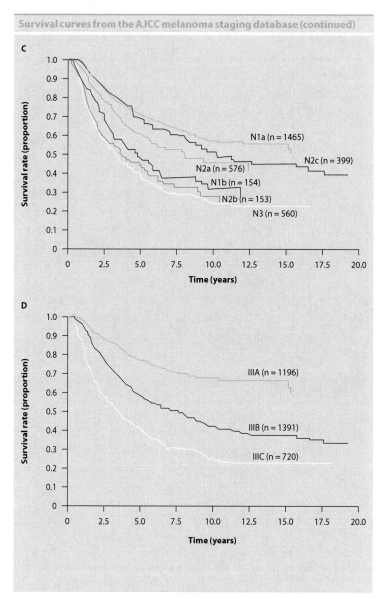

Figure 2.1 Survival curves from the AJCC melanoma staging database (continued).
The graphs above compare (A) T categories and (B) the stage groupings for stages I and II melanoma. For patients with stage III disease, survival curves are shown comparing (C) the different N categories and (D) the stage groupings. AJCC, American Joint Committee of Cancer; M, metastases; N, nodes; T, tumors. Reproduced with permission from Balch et al [12].

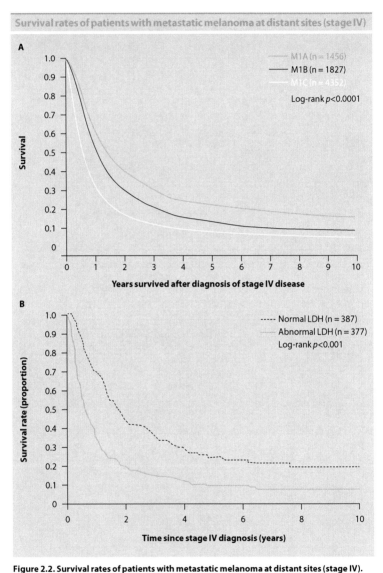

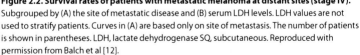

Figure 2.2. Survival rates of patients with metastatic melanoma at distant sites (stage IV).
Subgrouped by (A) the site of metastatic disease and (B) serum LDH levels. LDH values are not used to stratify patients. Curves in (A) are based only on site of metastasis. The number of patients is shown in parentheses. LDH, lactate dehydrogenase SQ, subcutaneous. Reproduced with permission from Balch et al [12].

Metastatic pathways and clinical course of melanoma

Metastases may arise from very small tumor masses that can circulate by two different metastatic pathways:

- **Lymphogenic** (mainly responsible for locoregional lymph node, in-transit, and satellite metastases), which accounts for around 80% of first dissemination; or
- **Hematogenic** (frequently responsible for distant metastases).

In about two-thirds of cutaneous melanoma cases, metastatic spread develops primarily as the local recurrence and/or locoregional metastases, while in about one-third of cases primary development of distant metastases is observed [15,18]. The majority of patients with metastases ($\approx$50%) develop regional lymph node metastases. In about 21% of patients, metastases appear as in-transit or satellite metastases [15,18,19] as, for example, shown in Figure 2.3.

Generally, time to appearance of first metastases is shorter for locoregional metastasis ($\approx$16 or 17 months) than for distant metastases ($\approx$24–30 months), irrespective of whether locoregional metastases

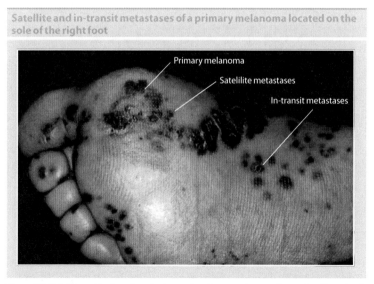

Satellite and in-transit metastases of a primary melanoma located on the sole of the right foot

Primary melanoma

Satelilite metastases

In-transit metastases

Figure 2.3 Satellite and in-transit metastases of a primary melanoma located on the sole of the right foot.

appeared first [15]. The risk of recurrence is highest within the first 3 years after melanoma diagnosis [19,20] (see Chapter 3, page 47).

Patients with distant metastatic disease have poor survival rates as depicted in the survival curves in Figure 2.2.

Late recurrences (ie, after ≥10 years after diagnosis) are described in rare cases (about 1–7%) and comprise patients with all stages of disease [21]. There are no specific predictors for the risk of late recurrence [20].

Take-home message

Metastatic spread occurs via the lymphogenic system in three quarters of affected patients leading to locoregional disease. Visceral dissemination occurs via the hematogenic system. Once melanoma has metastasized, survival rates are poor. Patients with distant metastases have a 10-year survival rate of only 5–20%.

References

1   Clark WH Jr, From L, Bernardino EA, Mihm MC. The histogenesis and biologic behavior of primary human malignant melanomas of the skin. *Cancer Res*. 1969;29:705-727.

2   Smoller BR, Histologic criteria for diagnosing primary cutaneous malignant melanoma. *Mod Pathol*. 2006;19(suppl 2):S34-S40.

3   Kaatsch P, Spix C, Katalinic A, Hentschel S. Malignes melanom der haut. In: Krebs in Deutschland 2007/2008. Berlin, Germany: Robert Koch-Institut; 2012:60-63.

4   Bradford PT, Goldstein AM, McMaster ML, Tucker MA. Acral lentiginous melanoma: incidence and survival patterns in the United States, 1986-2005. *Arch Dermatol*. 2009;145:427-434.

5   Glud M, Gniadecki R. MicroRNAs in the pathogenesis of malignant melanoma. *J Eur Acad Dermatol Venereol*. 2013;27:142-150.

6   Pollack LA, Li J, Berkowitz Z, et al. Melanoma survival in the United States, 1992 to 2005. *J Am Acad Dermatol*. 2011;65(5 suppl 1):S78-S86.

7   World Health Organization classification of tumours. International Agency for Research in Cancer. www.iarc.fr/en/publications/pdfs-online/pat-gen/bb6/BB6.pdf. Accessed June 20, 2013.

8   Chen LL, Jaimes N, Barker CA, Busam KJ, Marghoob AA. Desmoplastic melanoma: a review. *J Am Acad Dermatol*. 2013;68:825-833.

9   Curtin JA, Fridlyand J, Kageshita T, et al. Distinct sets of genetic alterations in melanoma. *N Engl J Med*. 2005;353:2135-2147.

10 Vidwans SJ, Flaherty KT, Fisher DE, Tenenbaum JM, Travers MD, Shrager J. A melanoma molecular disease model. *PLoS One*. 2011;6:e18257.

11 Curtin JA, Busam K, Pinkel D, Bastian BC. Somatic activation of KIT in distinct subtypes of melanoma. *J Clin Oncol*. 2006;24:4340-4346.

12 Balch CM, Gershenwald JE, Soong S-J, at al. Final version of 2009 AJCC melanoma staging and classification. *J Clin Oncol*. 2009;27:6199-6206.

13 Balch CM, Buzaid AC, Soong S-J, et al. Final version of the American Joint Committee on Cancer staging system for cutaneous melanoma. *J Clin Oncol*. 2001;19:3635-3648.

14 Individualized melanoma patient outcome prediction tools. American Joint Committee on Cancer. www.melanomaprognosis.org. Accessed June 20, 2013.

15 Meier F, Will S, Ellwanger U, et al. Metastatic pathways and time courses in the orderly progression of cutaneous melanoma. *Br J Dermatol.* 2002;147:62-70.

16 Gamel JW, George SL, Edwards MJ, Seigler HF. The long-term clinical course of patients with cutaneous melanoma. *Cancer.* 2002;95:1286-1293.

17 Liu W, Dowling JP, Murray WK, et al. Rate of growth in melanomas: characteristics and associations of rapidly growing melanomas. *Arch Dermatol.* 2006;142:1551-1558.

18 Soong S-J, Harrison RA, McCarthy WH, Urist MM, Balch CM. Factors affecting survival following local, regional, or distant recurrence from localized melanoma. *J Surg Oncol.* 1998;67:228-233.

19 Hofmann U, Szedlak M, Rittgen W, Jung EG, Schadendorf D. Primary staging and follow-up in melanoma patients – monocenter evaluation of methods, costs and patient survival. *Br J Cancer.* 2002;87:151-157.

20 Dicker TJ, Kavanagh GM, Herd RM, et al; Scottish Melanoma Group. A rational approach to melanoma follow-up in patients with primary cutaneous melanoma. *Br J Dermatol.* 1999;140:249-254.

21 Crowley NJ, Seigler HF. Late recurrence of malignant melanoma. Analysis of 168 patients. *Ann Surg.* 1990;212:173-177.

Chapter 3

Diagnosis, staging, and follow-up

Initial diagnosis
Visual and physical examination
Physical examination

After carefully taking the patient's medical history, their individual risk factors for melanoma should be assessed and evaluated (see Chapter 1, page 4). Patients should be asked if they have noticed the development of new lesions or changes in pre-existing ones.

For the detection of clinically suspicious lesions, a detailed visual examination comprising the entire skin (including the hairy scalp) as well as the visible parts of the oral and genital mucosa is required. The ABCD rule can serve as a clinical guideline to distinguish between benign and early malignant lesions during the examination with naked eye:

- A = Asymmetry in shape
- B = Border irregularity
- C = Color variation
- D = Diameter greater than 6 mm

Some authors have proposed E as additional criterion (Figure 3.1) and these Es are described: E = evolving, elevation, or enlargement. Furthermore, the term "evolving" seems particularly important since it includes changes over time with respect to size, shape, shades of color, surface features, or symptoms [1]. Any history regarding change in symptoms associated with pigmented lesions is important to render appropriate management decisions and to decrease thresholds for excision [2].

D. Schadendorf et al., *Handbook of Cutaneous Melanoma*,
DOI: 10.1007/978-1-908517-98-2_3, © Springer Healthcare 2013

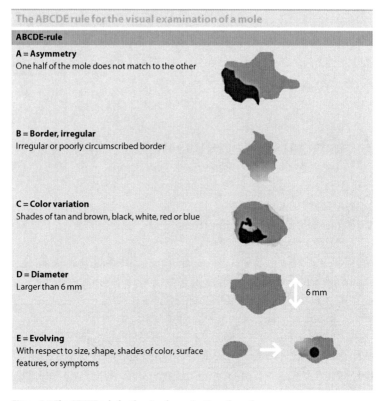

The ABCDE rule for the visual examination of a mole

ABCDE-rule

A = Asymmetry
One half of the mole does not match to the other

B = Border, irregular
Irregular or poorly circumscribed border

C = Color variation
Shades of tan and brown, black, white, red or blue

D = Diameter
Larger than 6 mm

6 mm

E = Evolving
With respect to size, shape, shades of color, surface features, or symptoms

Figure 3.1 The ABCDE rule for the visual examination of a mole.

It is important to note that not all melanomas present with all criteria and unrelated dermatological disorders, such as seborrheic keratosis and granuloma pyogenicum, can share some of those properties. Nevertheless, it is the combination of the ABCD(E) features (eg, ABC or A and D) that most often arouses suspicion of early melanoma in a melanocytic lesion [1].

Inspection of the pigmented lesions in the surrounding area of a suspicious lesion is important, particularly in the setting of multiple (dysplastic/atypical) nevi. Every individual has a unique clinic–dermoscopic patterns of nevi (ie, nevi in the same individual usually resemble one another). A lesion that looks different (so-called "ugly duckling sign") can be a helpful indicator for melanoma [2,3].

Once a clinically suspicious lesion has been detected and confirmed, the physical examination should also include palpation of the locoregional lymph nodes as well as the in-transit region (the area between the primary tumor and the first draining lymph node basin).

Dermoscopy

Dermoscopy is a useful tool for improving diagnostic accuracy, as it enhances melanoma detection and decreases the number of unnecessary excisions [4–6]. It is a noninvasive diagnostic technique and consists of a hand-held magnifier and a light source (Figure 3.2). To reduce surface light-scatter interference, an interface immersion fluid is applied between the transparent plate and the skin [4]. Other dermoscopes use polarized

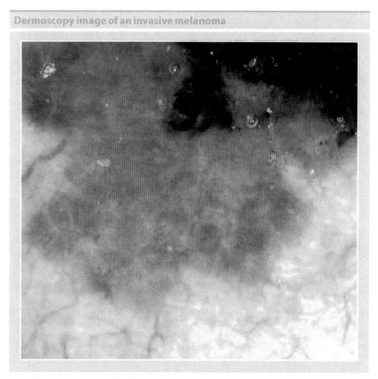

Dermoscopy image of an invasive melanoma

Figure 3.2 Dermoscopy image of an invasive melanoma. Regression zones are visible as milky red-white areas. Also note the different shades of brown pigmentation in the upper part of the image and the irregular blotches without a regular pigment network in the dark pigmented areas.

light and can be utilized without a liquid medium. Training and experience are mandatory for dermoscopy as the practice by untrained or less experienced examiners was demonstrated to be no better than clinical inspection without dermoscopy [4].

Multiple dermoscopic features have been described and several diagnostic approaches proposed, including the Menzies method, a 7-point checklist for dermoscopic scoring of atypical melanocytic lesions [2]. Table 3.1 summarizes dermoscopic features of melanoma that are of particular value [2].

Other complementary devices

Sequential digital dermoscopy is based on the same principles as conventional dermoscopy with the advantage of being able to save and digitally analyze images, thus allowing for an evaluation of skin changes over time. The Australian and New Zealand Clinical Practice Guidelines for the management of melanoma recommend the use of sequential digital dermoscopy to detect melanomas that lack clear dermoscopic features of melanoma [7].

Dermoscopic patterns for differentiation between benign melanocytic lesions and melanoma	
Dermoscopic pattern	**Description**
Atypical pigment network	Uneven thickness of the lines; presence of broad lines at the periphery of the lesion
Blue-whitish veil	Corresponds to infiltrates of melanophages below a thick epidermis with hypergranulosis
Atypical vascular pattern	Dotted and/or linear-irregular vessels and/or erythema within regression structures
Irregular streaks	Irregular lines at the periphery of the lesion that are not clearly combined with the pigment network
Irregular dots	Multiple black or brown dots, round to oval, irregularly distributed within the lesion
Irregular blotches	Black, dark brown, and/or gray structureless areas with asymmetric distribution within lesion
Regression	White scar-like depigmentation and/or blue pepper-like granules usually corresponding to a clinically flat part of the lesion

Table 3.1 Dermoscopic patterns for differentiation between benign melanocytic lesions and melanoma. Reproduced with permission from Malvehy et al [2].

Whole-body photography has shown to be useful for the early detection of melanomas and reducing the number of unnecessarily removed benign lesions, particularly in high-risk patients [8,9]. Other complementary devices of possible diagnostic benefit [10–13], which have not yet been widely established, include the following:

- Near-infrared spectroscopy
- Confocal laser scan microscopy
- Multiphoton laser tomography
- Optical coherence tomography

> *Take-home message*
> Physical examination includes the skin (including the hairy scalp) as well as all visible parts of the oral and genital mucosa. Suspicious and melanocytic lesions should be examined clinically, and several complementary devices exist for this purpose. Dermoscopy by trained and experienced examiners was shown to be of higher accuracy than examination by less experienced examiners or with the naked eye.

Biopsy

The clinical diagnosis should be confirmed by a timely skin biopsy, with the excision of the entire lesion as the recommended standard of care [14]. Accordingly, lesions suspicious of melanoma should be excised completely with a narrow lateral margin of approximately 2 mm or 3 mm of normal skin and vertically reaching into the subcutaneous fat tissue. Larger margins could cause disruption of local lymphatic vessels and consequently complicate the detection of the correct lymph nodes and therefore should be avoided [15]. Tangential excision by shave or partial excision is not generally recommended even if it is most likely not associated with an unfavorable prognosis [14], as deeper-lying melanoma deposits could remain in the skin impeding an accurate diagnosis of the tumor thickness and its horizontal size [16]. However, partial excision or punch-biopsy may be acceptable in large and widespread tumors in the face (Figure 3.3), mucosal, or acral locations [14,17].

Widespread lentigo maligna melanoma

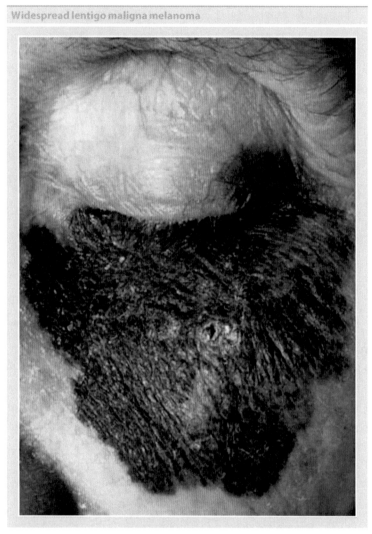

Figure 3.3 Widespread lentigo maligna melanoma. The tumor extends over the under and the upper lid of the left eye as well as over the left cheek.

Take-home message

Confirmation of melanoma is done by a timely skin biopsy. Excision of the entire lesion is the standard of care.

Pathology report

The specimen should be sent to a pathologist. The final diagnosis of melanoma is based on the histological examination of the entire lesion. A clinicopathological correlation should be made especially when there are large discrepancies between the clinical and the pathological diagnosis. The histological staging corresponds to the latest American Joint Committee of Cancer (AJCC) classification [18] (detailed tables of the AJCC classification: see Chapter 2, pages 18–19).

The pathology report should therefore contain the histological features required for a correct diagnosis and staging according to the 2009 AJCC classification [18–21] (Table 3.2) as these are correlated with the prognosis and possibly can influence subsequent therapy recommendations. According to the World Health Organization (WHO) classification, cutaneous melanoma is clinically and histopathologically divided into four major subtypes: superficial spreading melanoma, nodular melanoma, lentigo maligna melanoma, and acrolentiginous melanoma (for detailed descriptions, see Chapter 2) [22]. The localization of the primary lesion may be helpful for the definition of the subtype. It is advisable that the subtype is also mentioned in the pathology report, along with certain histopathologic specifics, such as presence/absence of regression

Essential components of the pathology report of primary melanoma	
Histologic feature	**Description**
Tumor thickness	Measured in mm from the bottom of the stratum corneum to the deepest lying tumor cell (Breslow)
Ulceration	Defined as discontinuation of the epidermis due to melanoma growth
Mitotic rate (in melanoma with a tumor thickness <1mm)	Defined as the number of mitoses/mm^2
	Determination is performed on hematoxylin-eosin slides; the evaluation of an area of 1 mm^2 is sufficient. Only mitoses located in the dermis should be considered [20,21]
Resection margins	R0: absence of microscopic residual disease
	R1: presence of microscopic residual disease

Table 3.2 Essential components of the pathology report of primary melanoma. Adapted from the Leitlinienprogramm Onkologie (Deutsche Krebsgesellschaft, Deutsche Krebshilfe, AWMF): Diagnostik, Therapie und Nachsorge des Melanoms Karzinoms, Kurzversion 1.1, AWMF Registrierungsnummer: 032-024OL, leitlinienprogramm-onkologie.de/Leitlinien.7.0.html [19], Garbe et al [20], and Piris et al [21].

zone, perineural invasion, and blood or lymph vessel infiltration (lymphangiosis melanoblastosa) [19]. Results of immunohistochemical stains (eg, S100 protein, HMB45, Melan-A/MART-1, vimentin, Ki67, CK) are used as adjuncts to distinguish between benign and malignant tumors and are helpful to discriminate epithelial-derived tumors from melanoma [23].

> *Take-home message*
> The pathology report of primary melanoma should include all histologic features required for a correct diagnosis and staging according to the 2009 AJCC classification as they are essential for the prognosis and subsequent therapeutic procedures.

Sentinel lymph node biopsy

Apart from tumor thickness, micrometastases in the sentinel lymph node are the most important factor for the prognosis of a primary melanoma [18]. Sentinel node biopsy is the acknowledged gold standard for the pathologic staging (N classification) of patients with melanoma who are at risk of clinically occult nodal metastases [24,25]. The indication for a sentinel lymph node biopsy depends on characteristics of the primary tumor (tumor thickness, mitotic rate, ulceration) and the individual patient's characteristics (eg, age, morbidity). The status of the sentinel node determines the tumor stage and influences both prognosis and further therapy (eg, complete lymphadenectomy for regional disease control when sentinel node was positive).

Indications for sentinel lymph node biopsy

The thickness of the primary tumor is the most important parameter for the indication of sentinel lymph node biopsy. As the risk of micrometastases in the sentinel node increases with tumor thickness, it is the general consensus to offer sentinel lymph node biopsy to patients with a primary tumor thickness above 1 mm and without any clinical evidence of locoregional or systemic disease [26]. In addition to the palpation of the locoregional lymph node basins, macroscopic lymph node involvement should be ruled out by preoperative ultrasound examination [19]. High-risk patients (patients with tumor thickness from 4 mm and with ulceration [stage IIC]) and patients with suspected locoregional and/or distant metastases should undergo further investigations prior to sentinel lymph node biopsy (see Chapter 4).

Apart from tumor thickness, several other factors have been described in the literature to be possibly correlated with sentinel node positivity [26,27]:

- ulceration [26,27]; and/or
- increased mitotic rate; and/or
- patient age at diagnosis <40 years [28].

If these factors are present, a sentinel lymph node biopsy should be considered and discussed also in patients with thinner melanomas (tumor thickness 0.75–1.00 mm) as recommended by the 2013 German Melanoma Guideline [19].

The more recent literature did not correlate regression of the primary tumor with micrometastases in the sentinel node [27,29]; in contrast, a lower rate of positive sentinel nodes was observed [26,29].

Before sentinel lymph node biopsy, the patient should be thoroughly informed about the potential risks versus the possible benefits of this invasive surgical procedure. Prognosis, possible therapeutic consequences (eg, subsequent complete lymph node dissection in case of positive sentinel lymph node, indication for adjuvant therapy) and course of the disease (eg, better local tumor control) should be taken into account when considering sentinel lymph node biopsy.

Take-home message

Sentinel lymph node biopsy is indicated:

- When tumor thickness is ≥1 mm; and
- When tumor thickness is 0.75–1 mm and other risk factors are present (eg, age <40 years, ulceration, and elevated mitotic rate).

Detection of the sentinel node

Sentinel node biopsy is a surgical procedure that can be performed with either local or general anesthesia. Perioperative complications occur in about 10% of patients and include seroma, infections, and wound separation, and in rare cases, functional deficits or nerve injuries [27,30].

The sentinel lymph node biopsy procedure is described in several publications and there is consensus among experts with regard to how the procedure should be performed [31,32]. Because of the risk of local disruption of lymphatic vessels, sentinel lymph node biopsy should occur prior to wide excision of the primary tumor. The sentinel node is defined as the first lymph node or group of lymph nodes in the locoregional lymphatic drainage region of the primary tumor.

The first step is lymphatic mapping with the aid of planar lymphoscintigraphy to identify the sentinel node(s) [33]. For this, a low-activity radioactive tracer substance (eg, Technetium-99m) is injected intracutaneously in close proximity to the area of the primary tumor (Figure 3.4).

Early dynamic lymphoscintigraphy images visualize the lymphatic channels. After accumulation of the tracer substance in the sentinel lymph node, the location of the sentinel lymph node can be determined using scintigraphic imaging and a gamma probe. The location is commonly marked on the patient's skin to facilitate the later detection of the sentinel lymph node(s) by the surgeon [31,32].

In areas where the correct localization of the sentinel node(s) with the gamma probe is more difficult due to the vicinity of the primary tumor and the sentinel lymph node (especially in the head and neck area), the use of a single photon emission computed tomography/computed tomography (SPECT/CT) prior to sentinel lymph node biopsy is advisable (Figure 3.5). It allows for a more precise positioning of the sentinel node(s) [33,34] and it has been shown that the use of SPECT/CT aided sentinel lymph node biopsy compared with sentinel lymph node biopsy alone is associated with a higher frequency of metastatic involvement and a better disease-free survival rate [35].

Intraoperative use of the gamma probe allows the operating physician to detect the exact location of the sentinel lymph node(s) in situ. All lymph nodes which have taken up the radionuclide should be considered as sentinel lymph nodes and therefore removed and histopathologically assessed [31]. Another detection technique is the use of blue dye (eg, methylene blue) or a combination of blue dye, scintigraphy, and the gamma probe. The blue dye can assist in the visual confirmation of lymphatic vessels and the sentinel lymph node(s) [33]. However, anaphylaxis, protracted

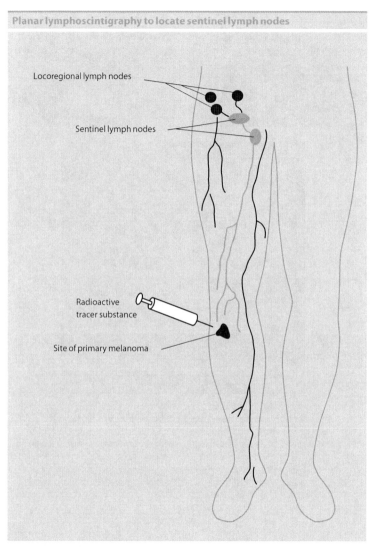

Figure 3.4 Planar lymphoscintigraphy to locate sentinel lymph nodes. Radioactive tracer substance is injected in the close proximity to the area of the primary tumor. The tracer is carried to the lymph nodes via the lymphatic channels. Lymph nodes that have taken up the radionuclide are considered as sentinel lymph nodes.

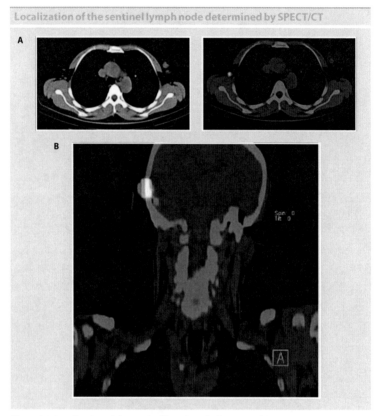

Figure 3.5 Localization of the sentinel lymph node determined by SPECT/CT. (A) Exact anatomic, two-dimensional localization of the sentinel lymph node determined by SPECT/ CT (right side) in the axillar area (bright area). (B) Exact anatomic , two-dimensional coronal localization of the sentinel lymph node determined by SPECT/CT: primary located on the right side of the head (bright area), two sentinel lymph nodes located on the right side of the neck (red areas). CT, computer tomography; SPECT, single photon emission computed tomography. Images courtesy of Dr J. Klode, Essen, Germany.

blue discoloration/tattooing, or cutaneous necrosis at the injection site [31] are adverse reactions that need to be considered.

> *Take-home message*
> Sentinel lymph nodes are marked with a radioactive tracer substance and located with the aid of lymphoscintigraphy (preoperatively) and a gamma probe (pre/intraoperatively). In special situations, SPECT/CT and/or blue dye can be helpful in the detection of sentinel lymph nodes particularly in the head and neck area.

Histopathologic work-up and report of sentinel nodes

Histopathologic work-up

Several different protocols exist for the histopathological work-up of sentinel lymph node(s) to detect small metastases [20,31]. It appears that examination of sections from only one tissue slice are not representative for the entire lymph node [36]. Therefore, various researchers describe techniques to examine increased numbers of slices and sections to optimize the detection rate for micrometastases [37].

Garbe and colleagues have proposed a compromise that describes the analysis of four tissue slices as a minimum requirement [20]. For very small lymph nodes, less than four may be sufficient. Staining should be performed with both hematoxylin-eosin and immunhistochemical methods. The most commonly used markers are HMB-45, S-100, and MelanA/MART-1, or a combination [20]. Frozen section analysis should not be used due to its low sensitivity. Polymerase chain reaction for the molecular detection of melanocytic markers was tested in studies, but was not found applicable in the clinical routine because of insufficient distinction between melanocytes and melanoma cells [38].

Histopathologic report

The following information should be given in the histopathological report of the sentinel lymph node(s) [19]:
- Evidence of melanocytes or melanoma cells
- Largest size of micrometastases (largest diameter)
- Number of metastatic sentinel lymph nodes
- Prognostically relevant parameters (in case of melanoma cells)

Various parameters have been described to have prognostic relevance and/or to be predictive of metastatic involvement of nonsentinel lymph nodes. These parameters should therefore be also mentioned. For a detailed description of the prognostic relevant parameters, see the section on complete lymph node dissection in Chapter 4 (page 63).

Diagnostic investigations

Imaging methods

Asymptomatic patients after diagnosis of primary melanoma

Based on the current literature, there is no evidence for the routine use of imaging investigations, such as CT, magnetic resonance imaging (MRI), chest X-ray, abdominal ultrasound, positron emission tomography (PET) or PET/CT, or skeletal scintigraphy, in asymptomatic patients following the diagnosis of a primary melanoma besides locoregional lymph node sonography (Figure 3.6) [39–43]. These examinations have the risk of false-positive findings, leading to uncertainty and fear in patients; abnormal lesions are initially suspected as metastatic disease and only later, after additional investigations or even surgery, confirmed to be nonmetastatic [42]. Upstaging and/or a change of the therapeutic plan because of the detection of clinically occult metastases is described only in very rare occasions in these low- to intermediate-risk tumor stages [39–43].

According to the 2009 AJCC staging system, prognosis of patients in melanoma stage IIC differs greatly from that in patients with stages IIA and IIB. Rate of recurrence for patients in stage IIC is around 44%, comparable to stage III B/C (51%) [44,45], and there is even an overlap in survival curves of patients in stages IIC and III [18]. The 2013 German Melanoma Guideline therefore recommends the same diagnostic procedures for stage IIC patients as for patients with suspected or histologically confirmed locoregional metastases [19].

Patients with locoregional and/or distant metastases

Radiographic imaging procedures in patients with both localized and advanced melanoma are important for determining the spread of metastatic tissue. The results of these examinations may have a considerable impact on prognosis and the therapy plan (see Chapters 4 and 5).

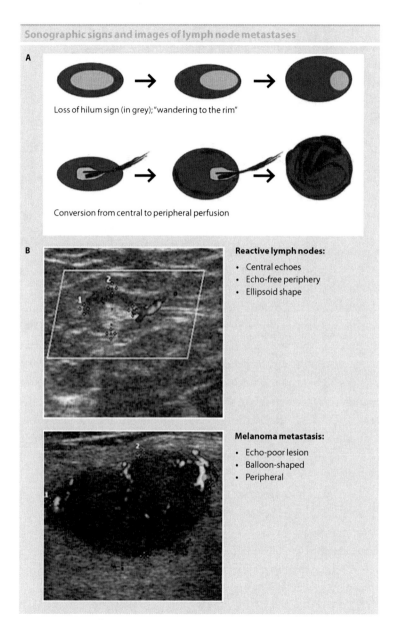

Sonographic signs and images of lymph node metastases

A

Loss of hilum sign (in grey); "wandering to the rim"

Conversion from central to peripheral perfusion

B

Reactive lymph nodes:
- Central echoes
- Echo-free periphery
- Ellipsoid shape

Melanoma metastasis:
- Echo-poor lesion
- Balloon-shaped
- Peripheral

Figure 3.6 Sonographic signs and images of lymph node metastases. (A) Sonographic signs of lymph node metastases. (B) Sonographic images: difference between reactive lymph nodes melanoma metastases in a lymph node. Images courtesy of Dr Christiane Voit, Berlin.

Examination of lymph nodes by midfrequency ultrasound (7.5–15 MHz) was shown to be of high accuracy [46], and is therefore the imaging method of choice to detect early locoregional lymph node metastases [40]. It is a low-cost, noninvasive technique without radiation exposure that is more precise than palpation alone [46]. The 2013 German Melanoma Guideline thus recommends the use of ultrasound in patients with stage IB or higher [19].

In case of micrometastatic disease, sentinel lymph node biopsy is the gold standard and cannot be replaced by lymph node ultrasound, as microscopic metastatic deposits are usually smaller than the resolution threshold of the ultrasound scanner [24,47]. However, lymph node sonography prior to sentinel node biopsy is useful to detect macroscopic lymph node metastases in the sentinel node and to possibly identify additional suspicious lymph nodes not marked as sentinel lymph nodes by lymphoscintigraphy [47].

Cross-sectional diagnostic technologies (PET/CT, MRI, CT) are the standard of care employed to exclude or confirm systemic disease [19], whereas conventional diagnostic methods, such as abdominal ultrasound or chest X-ray, have become less important. Among the cross-sectional diagnostic technologies, PET/CT (Figure 3.7) was shown to be superior to whole-body MRI or CT because of its high diagnostic accuracy [40], as it also shows areas with abnormal metabolic activity besides enabling precise lesions localization [48]. However, whole body MRI or CT are commonly used instead, due to the high costs of PET/CT in many countries.

Despite its high accuracy, PET/CT is not suitable for the detection of cerebral metastases because of the high physiological uptake of fluorodeoxyglucose by the brain [49]. MRI is the most precise imaging technique and the current gold standard for the detection of brain metastases [19,49]. Imaging procedures recommended at each disease stage are shown in Figure 3.8 [19].

PET/CT image of a patient with multiple distant metastatic disease

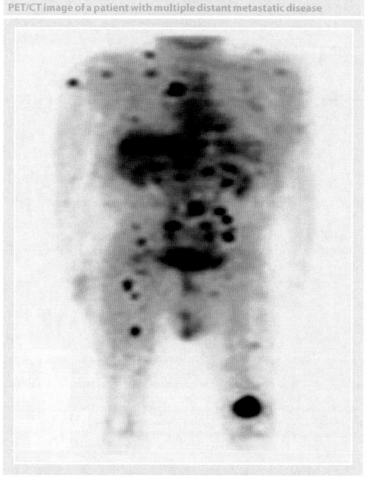

Figure 3.7 PET/CT image of a patient with multiple distant metastatic disease. CT, computer tomography; PET, positron emission tomography.

Take-home message

The method used for staging of patients with melanoma depends on the tumor stage. Conventional radiographic diagnostics, such as a chest X-ray or abdominal ultrasound, are no longer recommended; instead, cross-sectional diagnostic technologies (eg, cMRI and PET/CT, whole body MRI, or CT) are the standard of care in patients with metastatic disease.

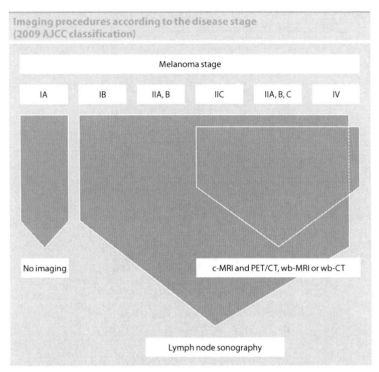

Figure 3.8 Imaging procedures according to the disease stage (2009 AJCC classification).
As recommended in the 2013 German Melanoma Guideline. AJCC, American Joint Committee
of Cancer; CT, computer tomography; MRI, magnetic resonance imaging; PET, positron
emission tomography; wb, whole body. Adapted from the Leitlinienprogramm Onkologie
(Deutsche Krebsgesellschaft, Deutsche Krebshilfe, AWMF): Diagnostik, Therapie und Nachsorge
des Melanoms Karzinoms, Kurzversion 1.1, AWMF Registrierungsnummer: 032-024OL,
leitlinienprogramm-onkologie.de/Leitlinien.7.0.html [19].

Biomarkers

Several biomarkers have been analyzed and published in the literature.
The most relevant and commonly used in melanoma are S100B protein
and lactate dehydrogenase (LDH).

S100B protein

S100B, a subunit of the S100 protein family, is a small, acidic calcium-
binding protein that is located in a variety of cells, including melanocytes and melanoma cells [50,51]. It has been shown that elevated levels
of S100B are significantly correlated with poorer survival [52]. This is

mainly relevant for patients with higher tumor stages, whereas the value of S100B in stage I and II is not entirely clear due to the lack of evidence [52,53]. Nevertheless, since it is a noninvasive and low-cost procedure it can also be determined in lower tumor stages.

Lactate dehydrogenase

LDH is a nonspecific serum marker but a valuable prognostic factor in stage IV disease. Studies have shown that survival deteriorates in patients with advanced melanoma as LDH levels increase [18,54]. The 2009 AJCC staging system requires the determination of the LDH serum level at the time stage IV disease is first documented. If the LDH level is elevated, patients should be assigned to M1c regardless of the site of their distant metastases [18].

In stage III patients with macrometastases, elevated LDH levels appear to be correlated with a worse prognosis, whereas this was not observed in stage III patients with micrometastases [55]. Therefore, LDH may serve as an additional prognostic marker in patients with locoregional macrometastases.

Take-home message

S100B and LDH are important tumor markers for melanoma. According to the 2009 AJCC classification, determination of serum LDH levels is required when patients enter stage IV disease.

Follow-up

Surveillance is an essential part of melanoma management as patients are at a high risk of disease recurrence or metastases. This is particularly important as effective therapies for melanoma have been emerging in recent years. Furthermore, patients with melanoma are likely to develop a second primary melanoma as well as other epithelial skin cancers [45]. Most guidelines recommend follow-up services for a period of 10 years or longer, some of them lifelong [45]. However, there is no clear international standard in view of duration, frequency of follow-up visits, or examinations at follow-up [44,45].

The risk of recurrence in patients with melanoma depends on the stage of disease. The AJCC classification respects important prognostic factors, such as tumor thickness, ulceration, and mitotic rate. While patients with thin primaries and without evidence of metastatic spread (stage IA) have a low risk of recurrence (about 5.2% as reported in Leiter et al [44]), patients in higher stages experience relapses significantly more frequently (eg, 44.3% in patients with IIC melanoma) [18,44]. Follow-up recommendations, such as in the 2013 German Melanoma Guideline, were developed on both the basis of the observed and calculated recurrence rates and the tumor stage [19]. Eighty percent of recurrences occur within the first 3 years following melanoma diagnosis [39,56], and the risk of recurrence stabilizes after 10 years [45,57]. A more intensive follow-up is therefore required in the first years after diagnosis. In rare cases (see Chapter 2), late recurrences of melanoma appear after 10 years [56], so patients should be educated to perform lifelong self-examinations [57].

Take-home message

The aims of follow-up are:

- To detect melanoma recurrence and metastases early; and/or
- To detect secondary melanoma as well as other epithelial skin cancers.

Because the risk of recurrence is the highest in the first 3 years after primary diagnosis, intensive follow-up (quarterly or semiannually) is required. The recommended duration of follow-up is 10 years.

References

1   Abbasi NR, Shaw HM, Rigel DS, et al. Early diagnosis of cutaneous melanoma: revisiting the ABCD criteria. *JAMA*. 2004;292:2771-2776.

2   Malvehy J, Puig S, Argenziano G, Marghoob AA, Soyer HP; International Dermoscopy Society Board. Dermoscopy report: proposal for standardization: results of a consensus meeting of the International Dermoscopy Society. *J Am Acad Dermatol*. 2007;57:84-95.

3   Grob JJ, Bonerandi JJ. The 'ugly duckling' sign: identification of the common characteristics of nevi in an individual as a basis for melanoma screening. *Arch Dermatol*. 1998;134:103-104.

4   Kittler H, Pehamberger H, Wolff K, Binder M. Diagnostic accuracy of dermoscopy. *Lancet Oncol*. 2002;3:159-165.

5   Bafounta M-L, Beauchet A, Aegerter P, Saiag P. Is dermoscopy (epiluminescence microscopy) useful for the diagnosis of melanoma? Results of a meta-analysis using techniques adapted to the evaluation of diagnostic tests. *Arch Dermatol*. 2001;137:1343-1350.

6 Vestergaard ME, Macaskill P, Holt PE, Menzies SW. Dermoscopy compared with naked eye examination for the diagnosis of primary melanoma: a meta-analysis of studies performed in a clinical setting. *Br J Dermatol*. 2008;159:669-676.

7 Australian Cancer Network Melanoma Guidelines Revision Working Party. Clinical Practice Guidelines for the Management of Melanoma in Australia and New Zealand: Evidence-Based Best Practice Guidelines. Wellington, New Zealand: Cancer Council Australia and Australian Cancer Network and the Sydney and New Zealand Guidelines Group; 2008.

8 Kelly JW, Yeatman JM, Regalia C, Mason G, Henham AP. A high incidence of melanoma found in patients with multiple dysplastic naevi by photographic surveillance. *Med J Aust*. 1997;167:191-194.

9 Feit NE, Dusza SW, Marghoob AA. Melanomas detected with the aid of total cutaneous photography. *Br J Dermatol*. 2004;150:706-714.

10 McIntosh LM, Summers R, Jackson M, et al. Towards non-invasive screening of skin lesions by near-infrared spectroscopy. *J Invest Dermatol*. 2001;116:175-181.

11 Langley RGB, Walsh N, Sutherland AE, et al. The diagnostic accuracy of in vivo confocal scanning laser microscopy compared to dermoscopy of benign and malignant melanocytic lesions: a prospective study. *Dermatology*. 2007;215:365-372.

12 Dimitrow E, Ziemer M, Koehler MJ, et al. Sensitivity and specificity of multiphoton laser tomography for in vivo and ex vivo diagnosis of malignant melanoma. *J Invest Dermatol*. 2009;129:1752-1758.

13 Gambichler T, Orlikov A, Vasa R, et al. In vivo optical coherence tomography of basal cell carcinoma. *J Dermatol Sci*. 2007;45:167-173.

14 Pflugfelder A, Weide B, Eigentler TK, et al. Incisional biopsy and melanoma prognosis: facts and controversies. *Clin Dermatol*. 2010;28:316-318.

15 Tran KT, Wright NA, Cockerell CJ. Biopsy of the pigmented lesion—when and how. *J Am Acad Dermatol*. 2008;59:852-871.

16 Witheiler DD, Cockerell CJ. Sensitivity of diagnosis of malignant melanoma: a clinicopathologic study with a critical assessment of biopsy techniques. *Exp Dermatol*. 1992;1:170-175.

17 Tadiparthi S, Panchani S, Iqbal A. Biopsy for malignant melanoma–are we following the guidelines? *Ann R Coll Surg Engl*. 2008;90:322-325.

18 Balch CM, Gershenwald JE, Soong S-J, et al. Final version of 2009 AJCC melanoma staging and classification. *J Clin Oncol*. 2009;27:6199-6206.

19 Malignes melanom: diagnostik, therapie und nachsorge. Arbeitsgemeinschaft der Wissenschaftlichen Medizinischen Fachgesellschaften (AWMF). www.awmf.org/leitlinien/detail/ll/032-024OL.html. Accessed June 20, 2013.

20 Garbe C, Eigentler TK, Bauer J, et al. Histopathological diagnostics of malignant melanoma in accordance with the recent AJCC classification 2009: review of the literature and recommendations for general practice. *J Dtsch Dermatol Ges*. 2011;9:690-699.

21 Piris A, Mihm MC Jr, Duncan LM. AJCC melanoma staging update: impact on dermatopathology practice and patient management. *J Cutan Pathol*. 2011;38:394-400.

22 World Health Organization classification of tumours. International Agency for Research in Cancer. www.iarc.fr/en/publications/pdfs-online/pat-gen/bb6/BB6.pdf. Accessed April 17, 2013.

23 Ohsie SJ, Sarantopoulos GP, Cochran AJ, Binder SW. Immunohistochemical characteristics of melanoma. *J Cutan Pathol*. 2008;35:433-444.

24 Sanki A, Scolyer RA, Thompson JF. Surgery for melanoma metastases of the gastrointestinal tract: indications and results. *Eur J Surg Oncol*. 2009;35:313-319.

25 Wong SL, Balch CM, Hurley P, et al. Sentinel lymph node biopsy for melanoma: American Society of Clinical Oncology and Society of Surgical Oncology joint clinical practice guideline. *J Clin Oncol*. 2012;30:2912-2918.

26 Testori A, De Salvo GL, Montesco MC, et al. Clinical considerations on sentinel node biopsy in melanoma from an Italian multicentric study on 1,313 patients (SOLISM-IMI). *Ann Surg Oncol.* 2009;16:2018-2027.

27 Kunte C, Geimer T, Baumert J, et al. Prognostic factors associated with sentinel lymph node positivity and effect of sentinel status on survival: an analysis of 1049 patients with cutaneous melanoma. *Melanoma Res.* 2010;20:330-337.

28 Kretschmer L, Starz H, Thoms K-M, et al. Age as a key factor influencing metastasizing patterns and disease-specific survival after sentinel lymph node biopsy for cutaneous melanoma. *Int J Cancer.* 2011;129:1435-1442.

29 Socrier Y, Lauwers-Cances V, Lamant L, et al. Histological regression in primary melanoma: not a predictor of sentinel lymph node metastasis in a cohort of 397 patients. *Br J Dermatol.* 2010;162:830-834.

30 Morton DL, Cochran AJ, Thompson JF, et al; Multicenter Selective Lymphadenectomy Trial Group. Sentinel node biopsy for early-stage melanoma: accuracy and morbidity in MSLT-I, an international multicenter trial. *Ann Surg.* 2005;242:302-313.

31 Chakera AH, Hesse B, Burak Z, et al. EANM-EORTC general recommendations for sentinel node diagnostics in melanoma. *Eur J Nucl Med Mol Imaging.* 2009;36:1713-1742.

32 Alazraki N, Glass EC, Castronovo F, Valdés Olmos RA, Podoloff D. Procedure guideline for lymphoscintigraphy and the use of intraoperative gamma probe for sentinel lymph node localization in melanoma of intermediate thickness 1.0. *J Nucl Med.* 2002;43:1414-1418.

33 Gershenwald JE, Ross MI. Sentinel-lymph-node biopsy for cutaneous melanoma. *N Engl J Med.* 2011;364:1738-1745.

34 Even-Sapir E, Lerman H, Lievshitz G, et al. Lymphoscintigraphy for sentinel node mapping using a hybrid SPECT/CT system. *J Nucl Med.* 2003;44:1413-1420.

35 Stoffels I, Scherag A, Klode J. SPECT/CT for sentinel lymph node detection in patients with melanoma – reply. *JAMA.* 2013;309:232-233.

36 van Akkooi ACJ, Spatz A, Eggermont AMM, Mihm M, Cook MG. Expert opinion in melanoma: the sentinel node; EORTC Melanoma Group recommendations on practical methodology of the measurement of the microanatomic location of metastases and metastatic tumour burden. *Eur J Cancer.* 2009;45:2736-2742.

37 Mitteldorf C, Bertsch HP, Zapf A, Neumann C, Kretschmer L. Cutting a sentinel lymph node into slices is the optimal first step for examination of sentinel lymph nodes in melanoma patients. *Mod Pathol.* 2009;22:1622-1627.

38 Gutzmer R, Kaspari M, Brodersen JP, et al. Specificity of tyrosinase and HMB45 PCR in the detection of melanoma metastases in sentinel lymph node biopsies. *Histopathology.* 2002;41:510-518.

39 Hofmann U, Szedlak M, Rittgen W, Jung EG, Schadendorf D. Primary staging and follow-up in melanoma patients – monocenter evaluation of methods, costs and patient survival. *Br J Cancer.* 2002;87:151-157.

40 Xing Y, Bronstein Y, Ross MI, et al. Contemporary diagnostic imaging modalities for the staging and surveillance of melanoma patients: a meta-analysis. *J Natl Cancer Inst.* 2011;103:129-142.

41 Hafner J, Hess Schmid M, Kempf W, et al. Baseline staging in cutaneous malignant melanoma. *Br J Dermatol.* 2004;150:677-686.

42 Sawyer A, McGoldrick RB, Mackey SP, Allan R, Powell B. Does staging computered tomography change management in thick malignant melanoma? *J Plast Reconstr Aesthet Surg.* 2009;62:453-456.

43 Yancovitz M, Finelt N, Warycha MA, et al. Role of radiologic imaging at the time of initial diagnosis of stage T1b-T3b melanoma. *Cancer.* 2007;110:1107-1114.

44 Francken AB, Accortt NA, Shaw HM, et al. Follow-up schedules after treatment for malignant melanoma. *Br J Surg.* 2008;95:1401-1407.

45 Leiter U, Buettner PG, Eigentler TK, et al. Hazard rates for recurrent and secondary cutaneous melanoma: an analysis of 33,384 patients in the German Central Malignant Melanoma Registry. *J Am Acad Dermatol.* 2012;66:37-45.

46 Bafounta M-L, Beauchet A, Chagnon S, Saiag P. Ultrasonography or palpation for detection of melanoma nodal invasion: a meta-analysis. *Lancet Oncol.* 2004;5:673-680.

47 Stoffels I, Dissemond J, Poeppel T, et al. Advantages of preoperative ultrasound in conjunction with lymphoscintigraphy in detecting malignant melanoma metastases in sentinel lymph nodes: a retrospective analysis in 221 patients with malignant melanoma AJCC Stages I and II. *J Eur Acad Dermatol Venereol.* 2012;26:79-85.

48 Strobel K, Dummer R, Husarik DB, Pérez Lago M, Hany TF, Steinert HC. High-risk melanoma: accuracy of FDG PET/CT with added CT morphologic information for detection of metastases. *Radiology.* 2007;244:566-574.

49 Aukema TS, Valdés Olmos RA, Korse CM, et al. Utility of FDG PET/CT and brain MRI in melanoma patients with increased serum S-100B level during follow-up. *Ann Surg Oncol.* 2010;17:1657-1661.

50 Cho KH, Hashimoto K, Taniguchi Y, Pietruk T, Zarbo RJ, An T. Immunohistochemical study of melanocytic nevus and malignant melanoma with monoclonal antibodies against S-100 subunits. *Cancer.* 1990;66:765-771.

51 Nakajima T, Watanabe S, Sato Y, Kameya T, Hirota T, Shimosato Y. An immunoperoxidase study of S-100 protein distribution in normal and neoplastic tissues. *Am J Surg Pathol.* 1982;6:715-727.

52 Mocellin S, Zavagno G, Nitti D. The prognostic value of serum S100B in patients with cutaneous melanoma: a meta-analysis. *Int J Cancer.* 2008;123:2370-2376.

53 Mårtenson ED, Hansson LO, Nilsson B, et al. Serum S-100B protein as a prognostic marker in malignant cutaneous melanoma. *J Clin Oncol.* 2001;19:824-831.

54 Agarwala SS, Keilholz U, Gilles E, et al. LDH correlation with survival in advanced melanoma from two large, randomised trials (Oblimersen GM301 and EORTC 18951). *Eur J Cancer.* 2009;45:1807-1814.

55 Nowecki ZI, Rutkowski P, Kulik J, Siedlecki JA, Ruka W. Molecular and biochemical testing in stage III melanoma: multimarker reverse transcriptase-polymerase chain reaction assay of lymph fluid after lymph node dissection and preoperative serum lactate dehydrogenase level. *Br J Dermatol.* 2008;159:597-605.

56 Dicker TJ, Kavanagh GM, Herd RM, et al; Scottish Melanoma Group. A rational approach to melanoma follow-up in patients with primary cutaneous melanoma. *Br J Dermatol.* 1999;140:249-254.

57 Murchie P, Hannaford PC, Wyke S, Nicolson MC, Campbell NC. Designing an integrated follow-up programme for people treated for cutaneous malignant melanoma: a practical application of the MRC framework for the design and evaluation of complex interventions to improve health. *Fam Pract.* 2007;24:283-292.

Chapter 4

Treatment of primary tumor and locoregional disease

Initial treatment of the primary tumor

Wide local excision

After the initial excision of the primary tumor with a narrow resection margin and pathologic confirmation of cutaneous melanoma (see Chapter 3), the subsequent standard treatment is wide surgical excision to remove melanoma cells that may be present in the adjacent tissue [1]. The pathological examination of the specimen should confirm the completeness of the tumor excision and check for satellite metastases, as surgery can be curative especially in tumors with low thicknesses and in the absence of metastatic spread and can reduce the risk of local recurrence [1,2].

Available data on the extent of wide local excision for the treatment of melanoma are not unequivocal, and there is ongoing discussion on the optimum resection margins. However, several studies and meta-analyses demonstrated that narrow excision margins are as safe as wide margins in the management of primary melanoma [2].

The recommendations for the extent of the radial surgical excision margins are based on the Breslow tumor thickness of the primary melanoma [1] and are listed in Table 4.1 [3]. The vertical excision depth should include the subcutaneous tissue down to, but not including, the muscular fascia (Figure 4.1) or the respective underlying structures, such as cartilage or muscle in areas without muscular fascias (eg, the face) [1,4].

D. Schadendorf et al., *Handbook of Cutaneous Melanoma*,
DOI: 10.1007/978-1-908517-98-2_4, © Springer Healthcare 2013

Recommended surgical excision margins according to the Breslow tumor thickness of the primary tumor

T-stage	Breslow tumor thickness (mm)	Safety margin (cm)
pTis	Not applicable	0.5
pT1, pT2	1 to ≤2	1
pT3, pT4	>2	2

Table 4.1 Recommended surgical excision margins according to the Breslow tumor thickness of the primary tumor. T, tumor. Adapted from Leitlinienprogramm Onkologie (Deutsche Krebsgesellschaft, Deutsche Krebshilfe, AWMF): Diagnostik, Therapie und Nachsorge des Melanoms Karzinoms, Kurzversion 1.1, AWMF Registrierungsnummer: 032-024OL, leitlinienprogramm-onkologie.de/Leitlinien.7.0.html [3].

Situs after wide local excision of a primary melanoma on the upper arm

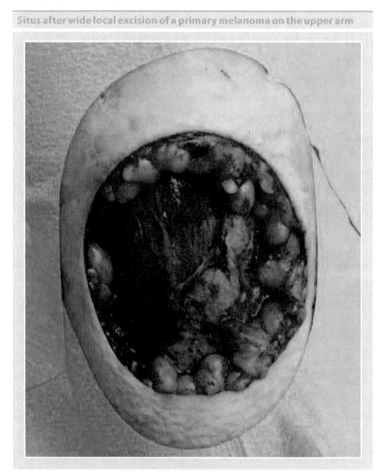

Figure 4.1 Situs after wide local excision of a primary melanoma on the upper arm. Note that excision was performed so that the muscular fascia can be seen.

Prior to the excision, the dimension of the safety margin needs to be determined, which can be done with the aid of a ruler (Figure 4.2). The corresponding distance of 0.5, 1, or 2 cm to all sides is measured and marked from the perimeter of the visible lesion, the scar, or edge of the ulcer, where the melanoma has previously been excised.

In anatomically restrained localizations, such as the face, digits, and genital area, there are no clear recommendations for optimal resection margin widths or depths. Deviating from the recommended safety margins may be inevitable because of the smaller area and the increased risk of cosmetic disfigurement or functional restrictions. To avoid an increased risk of local recurrences rates and to conserve tissue, micrographically controlled surgery (3D-histology) may be an appropriate technique in these cases [5]. First described by Moh in 1950 [6], who also lends his name to this procedure (Moh's surgery), and afterwards performed in modified ways by others, it allows for precise microscopic marginal control by in-depth examination of the entire circumference and surface area of the cut margin [7].

The decision on whether sentinel lymph node biopsy is indicated depends on the Breslow tumor thickness and on certain other risk factors, including ulceration, elevated mitotic rate, and patient age. Generally, sentinel lymph node biopsy is performed in the same session as the wide local excision. The indications and the procedure are described in detail in Chapter 3 (page 36).

Take-home message

Wide local excision with a safety margin is the recommended standard of care. Safety margins have a clear effect on the rates of local relapse, but not on overall survival. The wide excision margins are guided by the Breslow's tumor thickness; a full-thickness excision down to the muscular fascia is required. In physically and cosmetically restrained areas (eg, digits, face), where wide excision is not suitable, 3D-histology is recommended to preserve functionality.

Determination of the safety margin

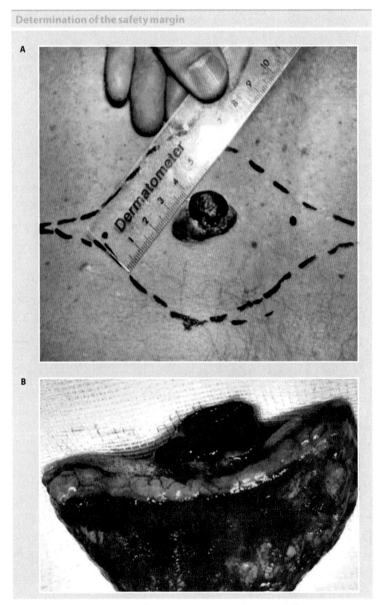

Figure 4.2 Determination of the safety margin. (A) 2 cm to all sides, with the aid of a ruler. (B) The vertical excision should include the all subcutaneous tissue down to the fascia.

Radiotherapy for primary tumor

Surgery is the only potentially curative procedure for primary cutaneous melanoma and is therefore the gold standard of treatment [1]. In cases where a surgical approach is not possible, either due to size and/or localization of the tumor or the patient's age or comorbidities, radiotherapy offers a viable treatment option with regard to locoregional tumor control [8,9].

Malignant melanoma has traditionally been considered a radioresistant neoplasm. However, several studies have shown that melanoma cells are not inherently radioresistant and are more sensitive to radiation than expected [8,9]. Radiotherapy may find application in patients with a widespread primary lentigo maligna melanoma of the face or neck (see Figure 3.3), in elderly patients with morbidities posing possible risk factors for surgical interventions, or postoperatively in patients with micro- or macroscopically positive resection margins ineligible for salvage surgery [8,9]. Another indication is desmoplastic melanoma, which has a high risk of recurrence [10]. Due to the lack of prospective, randomized, controlled studies, radiotherapy for the treatment of primary melanoma should be reserved for special situations, as outlined above. Patients need to be clearly informed about the potentially higher risk of local recurrences, related to possible remaining tumor cells in the skin, and long-term damages of the irradiated area.

Imiquimod

Imiquimod is an immunomodulator with antitumor and antiviral effects that causes inflammatory responses, such as erythema, swelling, and crusting. Several case reports and case series reported on successful treatment of melanomas in situ using topical imiquimod cream. This treatment may therefore be considered as an alternative for superficial, noninvasive melanomas in elderly patients who are ineligible for surgery. However, there have been no published randomized controlled trials, and results must be interpreted with caution due to the limited information from the reported cases [11].

Take-home message

Radiotherapy of the primary tumor and melanoma in situ offers a treatment option for locoregional tumor control in patients who are not eligible for salvage surgery. In cases of inoperable melanoma in situ, imiquimod can be considered, but confirmative data are limited.

Adjuvant therapy after excision of the primary tumor

Adjuvant treatment with interferon

Interferon (IFN; recombinant IFN-α2b and pegylated IFN) is the only approved therapy for the adjuvant treatment of melanoma in patients who underwent a complete surgical resection but are considered to be at high risk for relapse (pegylated IFN is approved only in the USA for stage III melanoma; IFN-α2b is approved in Europe and the USA for stage II and stage III melanoma). The rationale for the use of IFN is that by recruiting the host effector mechanisms, IFN eradicates possible subclinical micrometastases that may be the source of future disease recurrence [12].

Despite several randomized, controlled trials and meta-analyses on adjuvant treatment with IFN-α, the results and conclusions are not congruent and to some extent contradictory [13–15]. IFN-α was shown to provide a reproducible effect on disease-free survival time in patients with high-risk melanoma [13,16], but meta-analyses are needed to demonstrate an effect on overall survival. Recent reports suggest that high-risk patients (patients with ulcerated primary tumor and/or micrometastatic lymph node metastases) may benefit most from IFN therapy [17], although the biological basis of this observation is currently unclear.

The controversy around effects on survival may partially be due to the fact that studies differed with regard to the IFN type and/or treatment duration and were conducted in patients with different tumor stages. This is reflected by divergent recommendations in national guidelines. According to the 2008 Clinical Practice Guidelines for the Management of Melanoma in Australia and New Zealand, the use of IFN as an adjuvant treatment should be considered in patients with high-risk melanoma [18]. Other guidelines (eg, the 2006 guideline by the UK National Institute for Health and Care Excellence [NICE]) recommend that adjuvant IFN should only be given as part of a clinical trial [19].

Various IFN regiments can be used (Table 4.2) [20], and comparison between countries shows that different regimens are preferred by geographic location. Whereas low-dose IFN is the standard used in German-speaking countries of Europe (ie, Germany, Austria, Switzerland), high-dose IFN regimens are primarily used in the USA, where pegylated IFN has also gained acceptance in the last few years. Low-dose and intermediate-dose IFN are mainly used in southern European countries (ie, Italy, Spain, Greece), while some other countries (eg, Netherlands, Scandinavian countries) recommend the use of IFN only in clinical trials. However, recent meta-analyses strongly point to the fact that IFN duration and dosage is irrelevant for its effects on overall survival and relapse-free survival [13–15].

Side effects of IFN treatment have been frequently reported and affect various organ systems. Major acute adverse events are fatigue (70–100%) and flu-like symptoms (>80%), such as fever, myalgia, nausea, or vomiting, and these can appear up to 12 hours after administration. Symptoms generally taper off with the duration of the therapy [12]. The intensity of these symptoms can be reduced by premedication or symptomatic

Potential interferon regimens				
Type of regimen	**IFN dosage**	**Application route**	**Frequency (per week)**	**Length of treatment**
Low-dose IFN	$3 \, MU/m^2$	SC	3	18 months
Intermediate-dose IFN				
Induction	$10 \, MU/m^2$	IV	5	4 weeks
Maintenance	$10 \, MU/m^2$	SC	3	1 year
	$5 \, MU/m^2$	SC	3	2 years
High-dose IFN				
Induction	$20 \, MU/m^2$	IV	5	4 weeks
Maintenance	$10 \, MU/m^2$	SC	3	48 weeks
Pegylated IFN				
Induction	6 μg/kg body wt	SC	1	8 weeks
Maintenance	3 μg/kg body wt	SC	1	5 years

Table 4.2 Potential interferon regimens. IFN, interferon; IV, intravenous; MU, million units; SC, subcutaneously; wt, weight. Adapted from Jradi et al [20].

therapy with nonsteroidal anti-inflammatory drugs. Other main side effects include myelosuppresion, neuropsychiatric symptoms (especially depression), hepatotoxicity, cardiotoxicity, weight loss, and dysgeusia. Some autoimmune diseases (eg, psoriasis) that may be precipitated or exacerbated by IFN can persist throughout treatment but generally disappear after treatment completion. Overall, clinicians have to be aware that high-dose or pegylated IFN regimens are associated with significant toxicities [21,22]. Contraindications (especially neuropsychiatric and cardiac diseases) need to be ruled out before the initiation of treatment. Depending on the severity of the adverse events during therapy (determined by the Common Terminology Criteria for Adverse Events) dose reduction or discontinuation of therapy may be necessary [12]. Practical guidelines for the management of side effects are described in detail in a 2008 article by Hauschild et al [12].

The Common Terminology Criteria for Adverse Events (published by the National Cancer Institute; Cancer Therapy Evaluation Program) [23] is a detailed descriptive terminology for side effects caused by drugs; the Criteria can be utilized for adverse event reporting. A grading (severity) scale is provided for each adverse event term:

- Grade 1: mild adverse event
- Grade 2: moderate adverse event
- Grade 3: severe adverse event
- Grade 4: life-threatening or disabling adverse event
- Grade 5: death related to adverse event

Depending on the severity of the side effects, dose reduction or discontinuation of the applied agent can be required.

Take-home message

Recommendations for the use of adjuvant IFN in high-risk patients with melanoma vary by country. Due to the lack of other effective agents approved for the adjuvant treatment of melanoma, all high-risk patients should be informed about IFN treatment and thoroughly educated about the potential risks and loss in quality of life that can be associated with IFN. Alternatively, close follow-up and observation may be justified if these issues have been discussed in-depth with the patient.

Other adjuvant chemotherapies and immunotherapies

A variety of chemotherapeutic and immunomodulating agents have been evaluated as adjuvant therapies for high-risk patients with resected melanoma [24]. Chemotherapies were hypothesized to prevent the growth of tumor cells, reduce the volume of metastatic spread, and prolong survival. To date, no chemotherapeutic treatment was able to demonstrate a significant benefit on overall survival and/or disease-free survival. Therefore, IFN currently remains the only approved agent for the adjuvant treatment of melanoma.

The following agents have been explored:

- Monotherapy with **dacarbazine** compared with placebo did not show improved overall survival; in contrast, one study even demonstrated worse survival rates compared to the control group [25].
- **Levamisole**, an antihelminthic drug with immunomodulatory properties, was tested in patients with malignant melanoma in the 1980s, but failed to show any beneficial effects [26].
- **Bacille Calmette-Guerin** was initially explored as a live vaccine against tuberculosis [27]. It was also used in patients with melanoma in the 1970s, alone or in combination with other agents because of its observed immunomodulatory effects. However, neither the overall survival nor disease-free survival rate were significantly modified by this adjuvant treatment [28].
- Some practitioners, mainly in Europe, recommended **mistletoe plant extract** (*Viscum album*), as it is thought to play a role in immunomodulation. In a large prospective, randomized study, mistletoe therapy failed to demonstrate improved rates for overall survival and disease-free survival; instead, a nonsignificant negative influence on survival was observed [29].
- **Other immunostimulating agents** (*Corynebacterium parvum* and cytokines, such as interleukin-2 [IL-2], granulocyte macrophage colony-stimulating factor, and IFN-γ) did not show any therapeutic effect in prospective, randomized studies [20].
- **Vaccination therapies** were unsuccessful, and negative effects on survival were reported with some agents [20].

Take-home message

Apart from IFN, there are no other chemotherapies or immunomodulating agents approved for the adjuvant therapy of melanoma. Whenever possible, high-risk patients should be entered into randomized, controlled adjuvant melanoma trials to allow access to new agents.

Adjuvant surgical procedures

Adjuvant surgical procedures are also not recommended as a standard practice in the treatment of melanoma.

- While there is a general agreement that radical lymph node dissection is indicated in patients with histologically-proven or reliable suspicion of lymph node metastases, **elective lymph node dissection** (ie, the removal of lymph nodes without clinically detectable or histologically-proven regional metastases) currently cannot be used for the treatment of melanoma because of its lack of advantage on overall survival [30].
- Due to the high risk of side effects of **adjuvant isolated limb perfusion**, which can result in limb amputation in rare cases, it is not indicated in patients with melanoma. Although an advantage in local tumor control was demonstrated, no significant benefit was seen on survival or time to distant metastasis [31].

Take-home message

Adjuvant surgical procedures are not recommended in patients with melanoma.

Treatment of locoregional metastases

In patients with melanoma, the term locoregional metastases refers to local recurrences and in-transit, satellite, and lymph node metastases:

- **Local recurrence** refers to the reappearance of melanoma in the area or vicinity of a previously removed melanoma.
- **Satellite metastasis** is defined as the development of metastatic nodules within 2 cm of the primary tumor.
- **In-transit metastasis** develops in the metastatic drainage area from the primary tumor to the first regional lymph node basin [32].

Satellite and in-transit metastases are illustrated in Figure 4.3.

Surgical treatment

Complete lymph node dissection

Complete lymph node dissection, also referred to lymphadenectomy, is a surgical procedure in which as many lymph nodes as possible in the local area of the tumor are removed (Table 4.3) [3].

Patients with histologically-proven metastases or with reliable clinical suspicion of lymph node metastases (by palpation and/or lymph node sonography, magnetic resonance imaging [MRI], computer tomography [CT], or positron emission tomography [PET]/CT) should undergo complete lymph node dissection provided that they are free of distant metastatic spread. Initially, it was assumed that complete lymph node dissection was a potentially curative procedure [33]. However, some recent publications have shown that this surgical procedure has no influence on survival [34]. There are no published randomized controlled studies

Multiple satellites and in-transit metastases in the surrounding area of a previously removed melanoma on the head

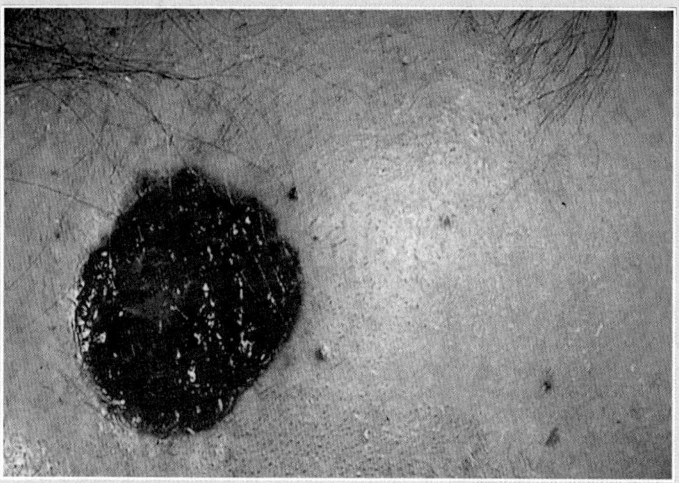

Figure 4.3 Multiple satellites and in-transit metastases in the surrounding area of a previously removed melanoma on the head. Image courtesy of Dr Axel Hauschild, Kiel, Germany.

Required extent of lymph node dissection as recommended by the 2013 German Melanoma Guideline

Area	Required extent	Extension
Head/neck	Modified radical neck dissection	Superficial (lateral) parotidectomy saving the facial nerve
		Posterolateral neck dissection (retroauricular and suboccipital lymph nodes, lateral neck triangle, parts of level II–IV dorsal of the internal jugular vein)
Axillae (upper extremity, trunk)	Level I–III, depending on the location of the primary tumor	
Inguinal (lower extremity, trunk)	Lymph nodes of the femoral triangle	Iliacal and obturator lymph nodes

Table 4.3 Required extent of lymph node dissection as recommended by the 2013 German Melanoma Guideline. Adapted from Leitlinienprogramm Onkologie (Deutsche Krebsgesellschaft, Deutsche Krebshilfe, AWMF): Diagnostik, Therapie und Nachsorge des Melanoms Karzinoms, Kurzversion 1.1, AWMF Registrierungsnummer: 032-024OL, leitlinienprogramm-onkologie.de/Leitlinien.7.0.html [3].

comparing patients who underwent complete lymph node dissection versus patients who did not. Therefore, complete lymph node dissection is still generally recommended, with the aim to render patients free of disease and provide effective regional control by lowering the risk of recurrence. In case of metastases in a lymph node basin that has been surgically resected, a second (radical) lymphadenectomy should be considered. Diagnostic imaging, such as CT, MRI, or PET/CT, are strongly recommended prior to surgery to rule out any further metastatic spread to a site other than the regional lymph nodes.

Lymph node dissection can cause significant morbidity. Perioperative complications occur in up to 46% of patients undergoing radical lymph node dissection [35,36]. The most common morbidities are seroma, which may require puncture and can become chronic, and chronic lymph edema [36]. Furthermore, patients may experience pain, wound infections (either postoperatively or following seroma puncture), hematoma, wound dehiscence, sepsis, or nerve injury [35–37].

Controversy remains regarding the management of patients with minimal tumor burden in the sentinel lymph node. Micrometastases (defined as metastases that were not detected by either palpation or

Micromorphometric features of tumor load possibly related to survival
• Largest diameter of metastatic deposit
• Subcapsular tumor infiltrative depth
• Number of positive sentinel lymph nodes (>3)
• Microanatomical location of tumor deposit within the node
• Capsular infiltration
• Extracapsular extension
• Tumor surface area

Table 4.4 Micromorphometric features of tumor load possibly related to survival.
Reproduced with permission from van Akkooi et al [39].

ultrasound) in the sentinel lymph node are an important prognostic factor for melanoma progression [38]. Tumor burden within the sentinel lymph node can vary. Various micromorphometric criteria (Table 4.4) [39] that influence prognosis and possibly predict positivity of further, nonsentinel lymph nodes were described and subsumed in different classifications (eg, Starz classification, Dewar criteria, Rotterdam criteria) [40], but agreement has not been reached [39], and it remains to be seen which classification is the most suitable. However, it is safe to say that prognosis worsens with increasing tumor load [39]. The combination of several parameters (especially the tumor burden and the localization of the micrometastases within the lymph node) predicts prognosis more precisely than a single parameter [41] and should be considered in the decision as to whether or not lymph node dissection should be performed.

Take-home message

Complete lymph node dissection is indicated in patients with metastases to the regional lymph nodes who are free of distant metastatic spread. The aim is to render patients free of disease and to provide effective regional control by lowering the risk of recurrence.

Prognosis decreases with increasing tumor burden of the sentinel lymph nodes. Micromorphometric pathology should be considered and discussed with the patient if a patient with a low tumor burden in the sentinel nodes can be spared a complete lymph node dissection.

Adjuvant radiotherapy after complete lymph node dissection

Surgery is the basic treatment modality for lymph node metastases. However, regional recurrences develop in 30–50% of patients after lymph node dissection [42]. Factors that are associated with regional recurrence include the following [4,43,44]:

- Large lymph nodes (>3 cm)
- Multiple positive lymph nodes (≥3)
- Presence of extracapsular extension

To date, postoperative radiotherapy has not demonstrated a significant impact on overall survival and is not routinely used in most institutions worldwide [43]. Therefore, there is a great disparity in the recommendations of the different national melanoma guidelines regarding radiotherapy. For example, the 2006 UK NICE guideline recommends adjuvant radiotherapy in patients who have undergone therapeutic lymph node dissection [19], in contrast with the 2005 French guideline, which states that no indication for an adjuvant radiotherapy exists [45].

However, adjuvant radiotherapy improves regional control in patients with melanoma at high risk for regional relapse after lymphadenectomy, compared with lymph node dissection alone [43]. Patients with the aforementioned risk factors can thus benefit from this intervention [43,44]. Also, patients with relapse in the lymph nodes after radical lymph node dissection may be appropriate candidates for adjuvant radiotherapy, as it is recommended in the 2013 German Melanoma Guideline [3].

Adjuvant radiotherapy is generally well-tolerated. The most common complication is lymphedema. The risk of lymphedema after lymph node dissection is potentiated by the use of radiotherapy [42]. To reduce the risk, conventional fractioning (≤2.5 Gy) and cumulative doses of 50–60 Gy are frequently used [43].

Take-home message

Adjuvant radiotherapy after lymph node dissection can improve local tumor control in patients with high risk for local recurrence, but has no effect on overall survival.

Surgical treatment of local recurrences and in-transit and satellite metastases

As for local recurrences, the approach for the treatment of satellite and/or in-transit metastases should be curative whenever feasible. Staging procedures to exclude distant metastases are necessary. In case of limited disease extension (limited local recurrence, isolated metastases, and a small number of nodules [eg, <10]), surgery is the method of choice and complete excision (both macro- and microscopically) should be attempted and verified by histopathologic resection margin control. When multiple and irresectable metastases occur, other modalities should be employed, as described in the next section.

> *Take-home message*
> Surgery is the standard of care in local recurrent and locoregional metastatic disease. Whenever possible local recurrences and in-transit and satellite metastases should be completely excised (R0) with curative approach.

Alternative local treatment options for unresectable in-transit and satellite metastases

Once metastatic melanoma becomes unresectable (eg, due to a high number of lesions, large tumors making a complete resection highly unlikely, or repetitive early recurrences), prognosis is unfavorable and systemic treatment options are limited [46,47]. In case of BRAF-inhibitor-sensitive BRAF mutation, patients should be offered BRAF-inhibitor treatment. Another treatment option is ipilimumab, but it has to be noted that ipilimumab has been approved as a first-line therapy only in the USA, whereas it is a second-line treatment option in Europe. Chemotherapy (eg, dacarbazine or fotemustine) can be offered to patients without relevant targetable mutations or who are not eligible for ipilimumab. However, neither mono- nor polychemotherapeutic regimens could demonstrate a significant benefit on overall survival to date. Whenever possible, patients should be entered into clinical trials that offer access to new treatments, which might possibly have an impact not only on the progression-free but also on overall survival. Systemtic therapy options are described in detail in Chapter 5.

Although a variety of local treatments are being used, there is no recommended standard of care for patients with skin and soft-tissue metastases [46]. Superior efficacy of one therapy over another has not been established yet.

The local application of drugs has the advantage of achieving high concentrations at the tumor site, leading to a therapeutic effect without severe side effects, as the systemic concentrations of the agents are generally low [46,47]. The local application of chemotherapeutic agents, especially in patients with fast-progressing disease can be combined with electroporation or hyperthermia, as it is done in electrochemotherapy and isolated limb perfusion, respectively. The potential advantages of each therapy have to be weighed against the toxicity of the treatment or the agents used, taking into account the individual situation of the patient and the general constitution.

Take-home message

All local treatment approaches (eg, electrochemotherapy and limb perfusion) have a great potential to improve local control but do not provide any overall survival benefit. Adverse events, quality of life issues, costs, and patient's wishes need to be balanced.

Immunotherapy

IL-2 was initially used as a high-dose immunotherapy in patients with melanoma and was approved in 1998 as a first-line treatment by the US Food and Drug Administration (FDA) [47]. In Europe, the systemic use of IL-2 is not approved and is not a standard treatment for patients with metastatic melanoma [4]. In contrast to the systemic use that frequently produces adverse events, including fever, chills, hypotension, cardiac arrhythmias, and others, the intratumoral application is generally well-tolerated [46,47], and several studies report regression of melanoma metastases after intratumoral IL-2 treatment. Intratumoral injections cause an inflammatory reaction at the site of injection with local swelling and erythema, inducing a selective necrosis of the tumor tissue. Frequent side effects are pain at the injection site, fever, flu-like symptoms, fatigue, and nausea [47]. Patients with stage III melanoma with cutaneous metastases can benefit from intratumoral IL-2, which may lead to complete remission (in approximately 60% of cases) and favorable long-term outcomes [46,47].

Since the late 1970s another immunomodulating agent, **dinitrochlorobenzene**, has been explored for the treatment of skin metastases of melanoma. It is an obligatory contact allergen, which is applied locally to sensitize skin in order to increase cytotoxic effects by inflammation [48,49]. Side effects include erythema, swelling, blistering and epidermolysis, ulceration, fever, nausea, and general malaise [48]. In publications, partial or complete remission rates up to 37–69% were reported [48,49].

IFN has been proposed to have immunomodulating and thus antiproliferative properties against melanoma cells [50]. Different IFN subtypes and different regimens have been used for the local treatment of skin metastases, but a dose-response curve could not be established. Therapy with intralesional IFN-α, IFN-α2b, and IFN-β achieve response rates up to 50% [50,51]. Due to a systemic effect, some patients experience side effects, such as flu-like symptoms, fever, headache, chills, myalgia, apathia, and fatigue. Granulocatopenia, an increase of liver enzymes were also observed [50,51].

While no significant benefit of **Bacille Calmette-Guerin** was observed in a postsurgical adjuvant therapy in patients with localized disease or as an addition to chemotherapeutic regimens in patients with metastatic disease, the intralesional application in patients with cutaneous metastases was associated with good response rates (complete response: 19%; partial response: 26%) [52].

Imiquimod, a synthetic imidazoquinoline amine, is usually used topically (5% cream) as an immune modulator with both antiviral and antitumor activities. Indications for topical imiquimod include anogenital warts, actinic keratosis, and basal cell carcinomas. The application of imiquimod for the treatment of cutaneous melanoma metastases might cause induction of melanoma-specific cytotoxic cells, leading to complete or partial remission of melanoma metastases in some patients [53].

Electrochemotherapy

Electrochemotherapy combines intralesional injections of low doses of a chemotherapeutic agent and local (percutaneous) application of electric pulses, which permeabilizes tumor cells (known as electroporation) and thus increases drug delivery into cells (Figure 4.4). Response rates of approximately 68% were observed in electrochemotherapy with cisplatin and bleomycin [54,55]. The major side effects of this therapy are pain due to the intratumoral injection of the agent and muscle spasms with myoclonia, which can be prevented by general or local anesthesia prior to the treatment procedure [55]. Other adverse events include erythema, edema, and necrosis [54,55]. The main advantage of this therapy is the reduced toxicity due to the low doses of drugs needed to achieve a tumor response [54].

Isolated limb perfusion and infusion

Isolated limb perfusion is a surgical technique that can result in partial or complete tumor remission on the treated extremity [56]. The circulation

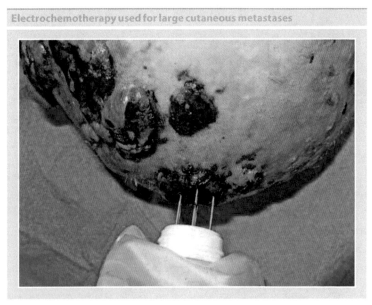

Figure 4.4 Electrochemotherapy used for large cutaneous metastases. Shown here on the patient's head. Image courtesy of Dr K.C. Kaehler, Kiel, Germany.

of an extremity is separated from the rest of the body with the aid of two tubes that are placed into the main artery and vein of the treated limb. A tourniquet proximal from the tubes prevents blood flow from the treated limb into the body. The chemotherapeutic agent is applied to the primary site via the arterial catheter and is circulated through the limb for a short period while systemic toxicity remains low (Figure 4.5) [56,57].

Isolated limb perfusion is performed under general anesthesia. Since 1969, hyperthermia has been added to isolated limb perfusion, as synergistic cytotoxicity of alkylating agents and heat is assumed [56]. Melphalan is the most commonly used single agent for isolated limb perfusion. More recently, the addition of tumor necrosis factor-α has been explored and was shown to provide better response rates than isolated limb perfusion with melphalan alone [58]. Possible complications of this treatment are mostly temporary and include erythema, edema, pain, nerve injury, wound infection, compartment syndrome, and rhabdomyolysis [59]. Long-term morbidity comprises lasting edema, neuropathy, muscle atrophy, limb malfunction, and venous thrombosis. In rare cases toxicity-related limb amputation may be required [59].

Isolated limb infusion offers another way to deliver drugs, such as melphalan locally. In contrast to isolated limb perfusion, it is a less invasive technique that does not require surgical incision because catheters are placed percutaneously in the artery and vein of the involved extremity. Therefore, general anesthesia is not needed and repeated treatments are possible. The lower rate of severe adverse events is advantageous and isolated limb infusion is generally well-tolerated. However, compared with isolated limb perfusion, complete and overall response rates of isolated limb infusion seem to be lower [60].

Both isolated limb perfusion and isolated limb infusion are not performed in all hospitals and require a high level of experience to achieve low complication rates. Currently, isolated limb infusion is mainly used in Australia, while isolated limb perfusion is the preferred treatment modality in most other countries.

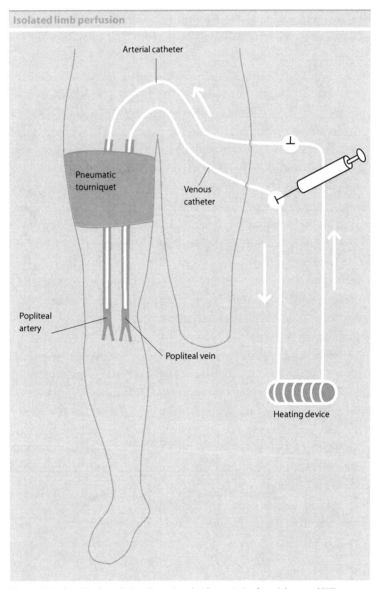

Figure 4.5 Isolated limb perfusion. Reproduced with permission from Ashton et al [57].

Cryosurgery and carbon dioxide laser

Other therapeutic approaches suitable for the palliation of locoregional cutaneous metastases are described in the literature, including cryosurgery and carbon dioxide laser. The latter uses continuous wave laser light that vaporizes the metastatic tissue, causing superficial burns (applied under local anesthesia). Laser therapy can be particularly effective in low-volume metastases [61].

Radiotherapy of locoregional metastases

Local radiotherapy was shown to have high response rates in patients with inoperable and locally advanced metastatic disease, and therefore offers another palliative treatment option for these patients [62,63].

Take-home message

If in-transit and satellite metastases are nonresectable, other therapeutic modalities can be considered, including the intralesional or topical application of immunomodulating agents, electrochemotherapy, isolated limb perfusion or infusion, laser therapy, cryosurgery, or radiotherapy. A decision on which treatment to use should be made after interdisciplinary tumor board discussions. A summary therapeutic options for locoregional metastases can be found in Figure 4.6 (see next page).

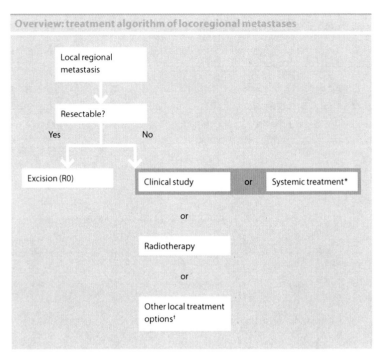

Figure 4.6 Overview: treatment algorithm of locoregional metastases. *First line: BRAF inhibitor in case of BRAF mutation, ipilimumab (USA), monochemotherapy; second line: ipilimumab (USA and Europe), polychemotherapy. †Electrochemotherapy, isolated limb perfusion/isolated limb infusion, cryosurgery, carbon dioxide laser, immunotherapy (topical application): interleukin 2, dinitrochlorobenzene, interferon, Bacille Calmette-Guerin, imiquimod.

References

1   Sladden MJ, Balch C, Barzilai DA, et al. Surgical excision margins for primary cutaneous melanoma. *Cochrane Database Syst Rev*. 2009;4:CD004835.
2   Mocellin S, Pasquali S, Nitti D. The impact of surgery on survival of patients with cutaneous melanoma: revisiting the role of primary tumor excision margins. *Ann Surg*. 2011;253:238-243.
3   Malignes melanom: diagnostik, therapie und nachsorge. Arbeitsgemeinschaft der Wissenschaftlichen Medizinischen Fachgesellschaften (AWMF). www.awmf.org/leitlinien/detail/ll/032-024OL.html. Accessed June 20, 2013.
4   Kenady DE, Brown BW, McBride CM. Excision of underlying fascia with a primary malignant melanoma: effect on recurrence and survival rates. *Surgery*. 1982;92:615-618.
5   Möhrle M. Micrographic controlled surgery (3D-histology) in cutaneous melanoma. *J Dtsch Dermatol Ges*. 2003:1:869-875.
6   Thomas RM, Amonette RA. Mohs micrographic surgery. Am Fam Physician. 1988;37:135-142.
7   Chang KH, Dufresne R Jr, Cruz A, Rogers GS. The operative management of melanoma: where does Mohs surgery fit in? *Dermatol Surg*. 2011;37:1069-1079.
8   Farshad A, Burg G, Panizzon R, Dummer R. A retrospective study of 150 patients with lentigo maligna and lentigo maligna melanoma and the efficacy of radiotherapy using Grenz or soft X-rays. *Br J Dermatol*. 2002;146:1042-1046.

9 Storper IS, Lee SP, Abemayor E, Juillard G. The role of radiation therapy in the treatment of head and neck cutaneous melanoma. *Am J Otolaryngol.* 1993;14:426-431.

10 Vongtama R, Safa A, Gallardo D, Calcaterra T, Juillard G. Efficacy of radiation therapy in the local control of desmoplastic malignant melanoma. *Head Neck.* 2003;25:423-428.

11 Ellis LZ, Cohen JL, High W, Stewart L. Melanoma in situ treated successfully using imiquimod after nonclearance with surgery: review of the literature. *Dermatol Surg.* 2012;38:937-946.

12 Hauschild A, Gogas H, Tarhini A, et al. Practical guidelines for the management of interferon-α-2b side effects in patients receiving adjuvant treatment for melanoma. *Cancer.* 2008;112:982-994.

13 Mocellin S, Pasquali S, Rossi CR, Nitti D. Interferon alpha adjuvant therapy in patients with high-risk melanoma: a systematic review and meta-analysis. *J Natl Cancer Inst.* 2010;102:493-501.

14 Wheatley K, Ives N, Hancock B, Gore M, Eggermont A, Suciu S. Does adjuvant interferon-α for high-risk melanoma provide a worthwhile benefit? A meta-analysis of the randomised trials. *Cancer Treat Rev.* 2003;29:241-252.

15 Pirard D, Heenen M, Melot C, Vereecken P. Interferon alpha as adjuvant postsurgical treatment of melanoma: a meta-analysis. *Dermatology.* 2004;208:43-48.

16 Eggermont AMM, Suciu S, Santinami M, et al; EORTC Melanoma Group. Adjuvant therapy with pegylated interferon alfa-2b versus observation alone in resected stage III melanoma: final results of EORTC 18991, a randomised phase III trial. *Lancet.* 2008;372:117-126.

17 Eggermont AMM, Suciu S, Testori A, et al. Ulceration and stage are predictive of interferon efficacy in melanoma: results of the phase III adjuvant trials EORTC 18952 and EORTC 18991. *Eur J Cancer.* 2012;48:218-225.

18 Australian Cancer Network Melanoma Guidelines Revision Working Party. Clinical Practice Guidelines for the Management of Melanoma in Australia and New Zealand: Evidence-Based Best Practice Guidelines. Wellington, New Zealand: Cancer Council Australia and Australian Cancer Network and the Sydney and New Zealand Guidelines Group; 2008.

19 National Institute for Health and Clinical Excellence. *Improving Outcomes for People with Skin Tumours including Melanoma: The Manual.* London, UK; 2006.

20 Jradi Z, Eigentler TK, Garbe C. Adjuvante therapie des malignen melanoms. *Arzneimitteltherapie.* 2012;30:46-52.

21 Kirkwood JM, Ibrahim JG, Sondak VK, et al. High- and low-dose interferon alfa-2b in high-risk melanoma: first analysis of intergroup trial E1690/S9111/C9190. *J Clin Oncol.* 2000;18:2444-2458.

22 Loquai C, Schmidtmann I, Beutel M, et al. Quality of life in melanoma patients during adjuvant treatment with pegylated interferon-α2b: patients' and doctors' views. *Eur J Dermatol.* 2011;21:976-984.

23 National Cancer Institute. Protocol Development. CTCAE v4.0 Open Comment Period. ctep. cancer.gov/protocolDevelopment/electronic_applications/ctc.htm. Last update March 20, 2013. Accessed June 20, 2013.

24 Veronesi U, Adamus J, Aubert C, et al. A randomized trial of adjuvant chemotherapy and immunotherapy in cutaneous melanoma. *N Engl J Med.* 1982;307:913-916.

25 Hill GJ 2nd, Moss SE, Golomb FM, et al. DTIC and combination therapy for melanoma: III. DTIC (NSC 45388) Surgical Adjuvant Study COG PROTOCOL 7040. *Cancer.* 1981;47:2556-2562.

26 Loutfi A, Shakr A, Jerry M, Hanley J, Shibata HR. Double blind randomized prospective trial of levamisole/placebo in stage I cutaneous malignant melanoma. *Clin Invest Med.* 1987;10:325-328.

27 Cayabyab MJ, Macovei L, Campos-Neto A. Current and novel approaches to vaccine development against tuberculosis. *Front Cell Infect Microbiol.* 2012;2:154.

28 Agarwala SS, Neuberg D, Park Y, Kirkwood JM. Mature results of a phase III randomized trial of bacillus Calmette-Guerin (BCG) versus observation and BCG plus dacarbazine versus BCG in the adjuvant therapy of American Joint Committee on Cancer Stage I-III melanoma (E1673): a trial of the Eastern Cooperative Oncology Group. *Cancer.* 2004;100:1692-1698.

29 Kleeberg UR, Suciu S, Bröcker EB, et al; EORTC Melanoma Group in cooperation with the German Cancer Society (DKG). Final results of the EORTC 18871/DKG 80-1 randomised phase III trial. rIFN-α2b versus rIFN-γ versus ISCADOR M® versus observation after surgery in melanoma patients with either high-risk primary (thickness >3 mm) or regional lymph node metastasis. *Eur J Cancer.* 2004;40:390-402.

30 Lens MB, Dawes M, Goodacre T, Newton-Bishop JA. Elective lymph node dissection in patients with melanoma: systematic review and meta-analysis of randomized controlled trials. *Arch Surg.* 2002;137:458-461.

31 Koops HS, Vaglini M, Suciu S, et al. Prophylactic isolated limb perfusion for localized, high-risk limb melanoma: results of a multicenter randomized phase III trial. European Organization for Research and Treatment of Cancer Malignant Melanoma Cooperative Group Protocol 18832, the World Health Organization Melanoma Program Trial 15, and the North American Perfusion Group Southwest Oncology Group-8593. *J Clin Oncol.* 1998;16:2906-2912.

32 Meier F, Will S, Ellwanger U, et al. Metastatic pathways and time courses in the orderly progression of cutaneous melanoma. *Br J Dermatol.* 2002;147:62-70.

33 Morton DL, Wanek L, Nizze JA, Elashoff RM, Wong JH. Improved long-term survival after lymphadenectomy of melanoma metastatic to regional nodes. Analysis of prognostic factors in 1134 patients from the John Wayne Cancer Clinic. *Ann Surg.* 1991;214:491-501.

34 van der Ploeg AP, van Akkooi AC, Rutkowski P, et al; European Organization for Research and Treatment of Cancer Melanoma Group. Prognosis in patients with sentinel node-positive melanoma without immediate completion lymph node dissection. *Br J Surg.* 2012;99:1396-1405.

35 Davis PG, Serpell JW, Kelly JW, Paul E. Axillary lymph node dissection for malignant melanoma. *ANZ J Surg.* 2011;81:462-466.

36 Ul-Mulk J, Hölmich LR. Lymph node dissection in patients with malignant melanoma is associated with high risk of morbidity. *Dan Med J.* 2012;59:A4441.

37 Starritt EC, Joseph D, McKinnon JG, Lo SK, de Wilt JHW, Thompson JF. Lymphedema after complete axillary node dissection for melanoma: assessment using a new, objective definition. *Ann Surg.* 2004;240:866-874.

38 Balch CM, Gershenwald JE, Soong S-J, et al. Final version of 2009 AJCC melanoma staging and classification. *J Clin Oncol.* 2009;27:6199-6206.

39 van Akkooi AC, et al. Expert opinion in melanoma: the sentinel node; EORTC Melanoma Group recommendations on practical methodology of the measurement of the microanatomic location of metastases and metastatic tumour burden. *Eur J Cancer.* 2009;45:2736-2742.

40 van der Ploeg IM, Kroon BBR, Antonini N, Valdés Olmos RA, Nieweg OE. Comparison of three micromorphometric pathology classifications of melanoma metastases in the sentinel node. *Ann Surg.* 2009;250:301-304.

41 Meier A, Satzger I, Völker B, Kapp A, Gutzmer R. Comparison of classification systems in melanoma sentinel lymph nodes—an analysis of 697 patients from a single center. *Cancer.* 2010;116:3178-3188.

42 Agrawal S, Kane JM III, Guadagnolo BA, Kraybill WG, Ballo MT. The benefits of adjuvant radiation therapy after therapeutic lymphadenectomy for clinically advanced, high-risk, lymph node-metastatic melanoma. *Cancer.* 2009;115:5836-5844.

43 Gojkovič-Horvat A, Jančer B, Blas M, et al. Adjuvant radiotherapy for palpable melanoma metastases to the groin: when to irradiate? *Int J Radiation Oncol Biol Phys.* 2011;83:310-316.

44 Strojan P, Jančer B, Čemažar M, Perme MP, Hočevar M. Melanoma metastases to the neck nodes: role of adjuvant irradiation. *Int J Radiation Oncol Biol Phys.* 2010;77:1039-1045.

45 Négrier S, Saiag P, Guillot B, et al; National Federation of Cancer Campaign Centers; French Dermatology Society. Guidelines for clinical practice: standards, options and recommendations 2005 for the management of adult patients exhibiting an M0 cutaneous melanoma, full report. National Federation of Cancer Campaign Centers. French Dermatology Society. Update of the 1995 Consensus Conference and the 1998 Standards, Options, and Recommendations. *Ann Dermatol Venereol.* 2005;132:10S3-10S85.

46 Radny P, Caroli UM, Bauer J, et al. Phase II trial of intralesional therapy with interleukin-2 in soft-tissue melanoma metastases. *Br J Cancer.* 2003;89:1620-1626.

47 Weide B, Eigentler TK, Pflugfelder A, et al. Survival after intratumoral interleukin-2 treatment of 72 melanoma patients and response upon the first chemotherapy during follow-up. *Cancer Immunol Immunother.* 2011;60:487-493.

48 Strobbe LJ, Hart AA, Rümke P, Israels SP, Nieweg OE, Kroon BB. Topical dinitrochlorobenzene combined with systemic dacarbazine in the treatment of recurrent melanoma. *Melanoma Res.* 1997;7:507-512.

49 Terheyden P, Kortüm A-K, Schulze H-J, et al. Chemoimmunotherapy for cutaneous melanoma with dacarbazine and epifocal contact sensitizers: results of a nationwide survey of the German Dermatologic Co-operative Oncology Group. *J Cancer Res Clin Oncol.* 2007;133:437-444.

50 Von Wussow P, Block B, Hartmann F, Deicher H. Intralesional interferon-alpha therapy in advanced malignant melanoma. *Cancer.* 1988;61:1071-1074.

51 Fierlbeck G, d'Hoedt B, Stroebel W, Stutte H, Bogenschütz O, Rassner G. Intralesional therapy of melanoma metastases with recombinant interferon-beta. *Hautarzt.* 1992;43:16-21.

52 Tan JK, Ho VC. Pooled analysis of the efficacy of bacille Calmette-Guerin (BCG) immunotherapy in malignant melanoma. *J Dermatol Surg Oncol.* 1993;19:985-990.

53 Wolf IH, Richtig E, Kopera D, Kerl H. Locoregional cutaneous metastases of malignant melanoma and their management. *Dermatol Surg.* 2004;30:244-247.

54 Sersa G, Štabuc B, Čemažar M, Miklavčič D, Rudolf Z. Electrochemotherapy with cisplatin: clinical experience in malignant melanoma patients. *Clin Cancer Res.* 2000;6:863-867.

55 Gaudy C, Richard MA, Folchetti G, Bonerandi JJ, Grob JJ. Randomized controlled study of electrochemotherapy in the local treatment of skin metastases of melanoma. *J Cutan Med Surgery.* 2006;10:115-121.

56 Cornett WR, McCall LM, Petersen RP, et al. Randomized multicenter trial of hyperthermic isolated limb perfusion with melphalan alone compared with melphalan plus tumor necrosis factor: American College of Surgeons Oncology Group Trial Z0020. *J Clin Oncol.* 2006;24:4196-4201.

57 Ashton KS. Nursing care of patients undergoing isolated limb procedures for recurrent melanoma of the extremity. *J Perianesth Nurs.* 2012;27:94-109.

58 Moreno-Ramirez D, de la Cruz-Merino L, Ferrandiz L, Villegas-Portero R, Nieto-Garcia A. Isolated limb perfusion for malignant melanoma: systematic review on effectiveness and safety. *Oncologist.* 2010;15:416-427.

59 Noorda EM, Takkenberg B, Vrouenraets BC, et al. Isolated limb perfusion prolongs the limb recurrence-free interval after several episodes of excisional surgery for locoregional recurrent melanoma. *Ann Surg Oncol.* 2004;11:491-499.

60 Raymond AK, Beasley GM, Broadwater G, et al. Current trends in regional therapy for melanoma: lessons learned from 225 regional chemotherapy treatments between 1995 and 2010 at a single institution. *J Am Coll Surg.* 2011;213:306-316.

61 Gimbel MI, Delman KA, Zager JS. Therapy for unresectable recurrent and in-transit extremity melanoma. *Cancer Control.* 2008;15:225-232.

62 Overgaard J, Gonzalez Gonzalez D, Hulshof MCCH, et al. Hyperthermia as an adjuvant to radiation therapy of recurrent or metastatic malignant melanoma. A multicentre randomized trial by the European Society for Hyperthermic Oncology. 1996. *Int J Hypertherm.* 2009;25:323-334.

63 Seegenschmiedt MH, Keilholz L, Altendorf-Hofmann A, et al. Palliative radiotherapy for recurrent and metastatic malignant melanoma: prognostic factors for tumor response and long-term outcome: a 20-year experience. *Int J Radiation Oncol Biol Phys.* 1999;44:607-618.

Chapter 5

Treatment of distant and irresectable metastatic disease

Patients who have distant metastatic disease (stage IV) should be discussed in interdisciplinary tumor boards with all relevant clinical partners (eg, oncologists, surgical oncologists, radiologists, radiation oncologists, and pathologists) on a regular basis. Decisions should be based on clinical history and most recent imaging results, which should be available to all decision makers. If necessary, additional specialists and surgeons should be involved. Pathologic confirmation of disease and results of molecular pathologic mutational testing of *BRAF* is required and should be performed at the beginning of stage IIIB. If *BRAF* mutational analysis is negative, the tumor should be analyzed for *NRAS* mutations to allow possible inclusion into clinical studies. Mucosal and acral lentiginous-derived melanomas should be tested for *c-KIT* mutations where these mutations are primarily found. Staging of patients with metastatic melanoma is routinely repeated every 6–12 weeks, depending on clinical parameters, symptoms, and the therapeutic option chosen.

Surgical therapy of distant metastases

Surgical resection is considered the therapeutic option of choice if all distant metastases are resectable and complete resection with no residual disease (R0) can be reached safely. Although some progress in the medical treatment of metastatic melanoma has recently been achieved, advanced melanoma is still an incurable disease and a surgical approach should also be considered.

D. Schadendorf et al., *Handbook of Cutaneous Melanoma*, DOI: 10.1007/978-1-908517-98-2_5, © Springer Healthcare 2013

Surgical treatment of distant metastases is appropriate if functional deficits can be avoided. Single-organ involvement (confirmed by magnetic resonance imaging [MRI], positron emission tomography [PET], or computer tomography [CT]) [1,2], low number of metastases, and long progression-free survival are prognostically good indicators, and may be helpful in the deciding whether to perform complete tumor resection [1–3]. The site of initial metastasis is another factor, as the collective analysis of the systemic treatment of distant metastases shows that patients with skin and subcutaneous metastases have a greater chance of survival than patients with lung or visceral metastases [3,4].

As tumor biology and growth kinetics are usually the most predominant prognostic factors, an initial wait-and-see approach can be applied after informing the patient. Similarly, first staging after systemic medical therapy allows for distinguishing whether a limited tumor spread at first diagnosis of stage IV is the beginning of a rapidly developing tumor dissemination. Based on the authors' own experience, it is advisable to restage a patient with uncertain tumor dynamics after 6–12 weeks in order to estimate the rate of tumor growth and spread before deciding on surgery of visceral organs.

There are currently no published randomized studies evaluating the benefit of surgical resections in the treatment of distant metastases of melanoma. The only publicly-available prospective data set was presented by Morton et al at the American Society of Clinical Oncology annual meeting in 2007, and included patients with stage IV melanoma who achieved a state of "no evidence of disease" after surgical intervention of distant metastases. This carefully selected patient population achieved a 5-year survival rate of around 40% [5]. Results of several retrospective cohort studies regarding the resection of solitary metastases in different organs (eg, lung [1,3], skin [3], bone [3], visceral organs, including liver and intestine [3,6–8], and adrenal gland [9]) indicate, in summary, that patients who underwent complete resection have better chances of survival compared with patients with incomplete or no resection.

Palliative operations can be performed for the relief and prevention of symptoms in the context of known, incurable distant disease [7]. Metastases can cause a variety of symptoms, such as bleeding, anemia, pain, extremity weakness, or paresthesia related to compression of the spinal cord by a metastasis. Metastatic disease in the abdomen can result in life-threatening small bowel obstruction or anemia [10]. Retrospective studies have shown that a high percentage of patients with symptoms had relief after surgical removal of the metastatic lesion [7,10].

Surgical therapy of brain metastases

Brain metastases (Figure 5.1) are the most common cause of death in patients with metastatic melanoma. They pose a major therapeutic problem, and can manifest with a variety of symptoms [11].

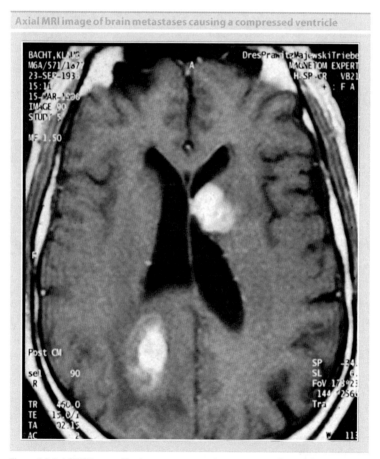

Figure 5.1 Axial MRI image of brain metastases causing a compressed ventricle.
MRI, magnetic resonance imaging.

Neurosurgical resection is recommended for patients with metastatic melanoma of the brain in cases of single and surgically accessible brain metastasis without extracranial metastatic spread and if the patient is in a good general condition [12–15].

Acute symptoms caused by brain metastases, including nausea, headache, acute bleeding, organic brain syndrome, convulsive attacks, or facial nerve paralysis, should lead to an interdisciplinary discussion as to whether neurosurgery should be considered. In clinically symptomatic brain metastases with increased intracranial pressure, whether or not to begin immediate surgical decompression for symptom control should take into account the patient's general prognosis, and patients may derive a significant palliative effect from such surgery [15].

Radiotherapy is another treatment option for brain metastases, and is described in the next sections (see page 83).

Take-home message

If surgery is feasible in cases of singular metastasis, it should be considered as the method of choice to achieve R0. Knowledge of tumor kinetics and dynamics, including the number and distribution of metastases, is helpful to select those patients who might benefit most from a surgical intervention.

In every palliative situation, the aim of the surgical intervention is a relief of symptoms and a better quality of life for the patient.

Radiotherapy of distant metastases

In the case of distant metastases, which are inoperable due to number, size, or localization, radiotherapy may be performed with the aim of improving quality of life, relieving symptoms, avoiding pain, and improving the local tumor control with no impact on overall survival [16,17].

The currently available data on the indication of radiation therapy in stage IV malignant melanoma (distant metastases) are poor, and there are no randomized multicenter studies on this subject. However, the idea that melanomas are basically insensitive to radiation, first put forth in the 1930s, cannot be maintained according to the available data.

Mainly retrospective cohort studies focus on radiotherapy of distant soft tissue metastases (skin, subcutaneous, and lymph nodes) [18], distant metastases of other localizations, such as the lung and liver [17,19], and skeletal metastases [20]. High response rates (up to 40–97%; partial and complete remission) and good palliative effects were described with radiotherapy with a cumulative dose of 30–40 Gy [17–19]. Response to radiotherapy is critically dependent on the size of metastasis, with an increased radioresistance with increasing volume [18,21].

The symptoms of spinal cord compression due to metastatic melanoma are particularly treatable with radiotherapy and stereotactic radiation, with an up to 85% improvement rate [20]. In cases of painful osseous metastases and/or risk of fracture, radiotherapy demonstrated a significant palliative effect with regard to pain reduction in nearly 70% of cases [22–24]. However, irradiation of asymptomatic metastases and metastases that are not destabilizing is not recommended.

> *Take-home message*
> Radiotherapy of distant metastases should be considered in order to achieve local tumor control and/or palliation. Response to radiation is inversely correlated with tumor volume.

Radiotherapy of brain metastases

Patients with brain metastases may be offered radiotherapy, with either stereotactic methods or conventional whole-brain radiotherapy [14]. In contrast to the whole brain radiation, stereotactic radiation precisely delivers radiation only to the metastasis.

Limited brain metastases should be irradiated with stereotactic single-dose radiation with the aim of improving the local tumor control, which can possibly extend survival [13,14]. Results from one of the largest analyses, by Eigentler et al, suggest a positive effect only in patients with singular or solitary brain metastasis. Median survival was significantly better for local therapy (at 9 vs 6 months), which means stereotactic single-dose radiation or surgery (complete resection), than whole-brain radiation and/or chemotherapy. This statistical difference between stereotactic single-dose radiation therapy and whole-brain radiation therapy diminished when patients with up to three brain metastases were included in the analysis [13]. Palliative whole brain radiotherapy should be offered for multiple symptomatic brain metastases with the aim of symptom relief if the patient is sufficiently fit for the treatment and life expectancy is longer than 3 months [11,12,14].

Detailed dosing recommendations for either stereotactic single-dose radiation therapy or for whole-brain radiation therapy that would be specific for the treatment of melanoma metastases currently do not exist. Additional whole-brain radiation therapy after neurosurgical intervention does not significantly improve survival rates [14,15].

Take-home message

In case of brain metastases, two treatment options are available:

- Stereotactic radiotherapy (single metastasis, no extracranial metastatic spread)
- Whole-brain radiotherapy (multiple symptomatic metastases)

No study to date has been designed to compare neurosurgery directly to stereotactic single-dose radiation. Therefore, no clear recommendation regarding the choice of therapy to achieve best local tumor control can be given.

Radiotherapy: fractionation

Therapy decisions in a palliative situation should always aim to consider individual patient requirements, avoid side effects, and reduce the treatment period. As conventional fractionation schemes show the same efficacy of local tumor control as higher single doses (>3 Gy) [16,25,26], patients with a relatively favorable prognosis and a life expectancy of more than 1 year should be irradiated with lower doses (1.8 to 2.0 Gy per fraction) to avoid long-term side effects (eg, atrophy, pigmentation, hair loss, telangiectasia, ulceration), as recommended in the 2013 German Melanoma Guideline [12].

Take-home message

The fraction size had no influence on the effectiveness of radiotherapy, so lower single doses are advisable to avoid long-term side effects. The cumulative dose of radiotherapy should reach ≥30 Gy.

Treatment of metastases in special localizations

Drug therapy of bone metastases

Bone metastases can cause such problems as persistent or intermittent pain, fractures, spinal cord compression, and hypercalcemia. Correspondingly, bone metastases can reduce quality of life and increase morbidity [27]. Therapy should start as soon as bone metastases are detected. Recommended pharmacologic treatment for patients with bone metastases is listed in Table 5.1 [12]. Oral and intravenous application of bisphosphonates (eg, ibandronate, pamidronate, risedronate, zoledronate) are comparable with regard to efficacy [12].

Intravenous administration is preferential if a rapid effect is necessary. Denosumab is another treatment option, which is not part of the family of bisphosphonate due to its different mode of action. It is a monoclonal antibody with high affinity for RANKL (receptor activator of nuclear factor kappa-B ligand).

For patients with a creatinine clearance above 60 mL/min, no adjustment of dosage, infusion time, and therapy interval is required. In patients with a creatinine clearance below 30 mL/min or in dialysis-dependent patients, periodic monitoring of calcium levels to rule out hypocalcemia is recommended. Supplementation with a minimum of 500 mg calcium and 400 IU vitamin D is recommended independently of treatment choice, except in the case of hypercalcemia [12,28]. The treatment, adapted to the individual course of the disease, should be continued for as long as possible.

Recommended pharmacological treatment for patients with bone metastases		
Drug	**Dosage**	**Dose regimen**
Denosumab	120 mg SC	Every 4 weeks
Pamidronate	90 mg IV	Infusion time: minimum of 2 hours; every 3 to 4 weeks
Zoledronate	4 mg IV	Infusion time: 15 min; every 3 to 4 weeks
Ibandronate	6 mg IV	Infusion time: 15 min; every 3 to 4 weeks
Ibandronate	50 mg orally	Daily

Table 5.1 Recommended pharmacological treatment for patients with bone metastases.
IV, intravenous; SC, subcutaneous. Reproduced with permission from Leitlinienprogramm Onkologie (Deutsche Krebsgesellschaft, Deutsche Krebshilfe, AWMF): Diagnostik, Therapie und Nachsorge des Melanoms Karzinoms, Kurzversion 1.1, AWMF Registrierungsnummer: 032-024OL, leitlinienprogramm-onkologie.de/Leitlinien.7.0.html [12].

An osteonecrosis of the jaw is a rare (<2%) but potentially severe adverse reaction to bone-modifying agents. All patients should undergo dental or surgical examinations of the jaw before therapy initiation with bisphosphonates or denosumab. Event rates for osteonecrosis of the jaw can be reduced by pretherapeutic mouth cavity sanitation. Optimal oral hygiene is important and surgery on the jaw bone or periosteum under bisphosphonates or denosumab therapy should be avoided, and if necessary only done under prolonged perioperative systemic antibiotic treatment [12,28].

> *Take-home message*
> Patients with bone metastases should receive bisphosphonates or the RANKL inhibitor denosumab. Due to the risk of osteonecrosis of the jaw that can be caused by bisphosphonates and denosumab, dental or surgical examinations of the jaw and should take place prior to treatment initiation. Monitoring of calcium levels and creatinine clearance before and during therapy is also required.

Localized therapeutic measures for liver metastases

Liver metastases (Figure 5.2) are observed in approximately 40% of all patients with visceral metastases. In ocular melanoma, liver metastases occur even more frequently than in cutaneous melanoma due to the lack of lymphatic drainage of the eye. Besides surgery (considered in case of limited disease if an R0 excision can be reached [8,29]), various localized therapeutic measures exist for patients who are otherwise free of metastases (Table 5.2) [12,30–41]. It must be noted that improvement in overall survival has not been proven yet for these strategies, which have been tested in cohort studies with retrospective designs and a mostly small number of patients. Localized therapeutic measures have been developed, as effective systemic therapies for melanoma have been unavailable [30]. Response rates (partial and complete response) for the different localized methods have been similar: 16–38% for hepatic intra-arterial chemotherapy [31–33] and 37–70% for isolated hepatic perfusion [34–37].

Liver metastases derive about 80% of their blood supply from the hepatic artery, while the liver parenchyma is mainly perfused via the

Axial MRI image of liver metastases

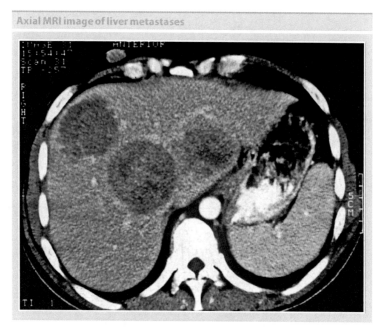

Figure 5.2 Axial MRI image of liver metastases. MRI, magnetic resonance imaging.

portal venous system [30,31]. Intrahepatic chemotherapy, chemoembolization, and selective internal radiotherapy were developed based on the advantage of this dual blood supply, which can help to spare normal hepatic tissue and minimize systemic toxicity [30,31]. Compared to isolated hepatic perfusion, laparotomy is not necessary and femoral artery catheterization is used instead [31].

Take-home message

Ablation, infusion/perfusion, and embolization strategies demonstrated clinical responses in small studies and can be considered in patients when complete surgical treatment is not feasible. However, data available for cutaneous melanoma are restricted and improvement in overall survival was not shown. Now that effective systemic therapies with benefit to overall survival are available (eg, *BRAF* inhibitors, ipilimumab), patients should primarily be considered for systemic therapies.

Procedure	Description
Radiofrequency ablation	Radiofrequency ablation is a method that utilizes heat to ablate tumor cells. Radiofrequency electrodes can be placed via open laparotomy, by laparoscopic surgery, or percutaneously with the aid of CT, MRI, or ultrasound [38,39]. Other methods work similarly but use laser beam, microwaves, or focused ultrasound energy [12].
Isolated hepatic perfusion	Laparotomy and subsequent mobilization of the liver are required to temporarily isolate the liver's blood supply with the use of two catheters. Thus, high dosages of anticancer drugs can be delivered to the liver only. Most of the available clinical experience and evidence relates to isolated hepatic perfusion with melphalan (± TNF-α) [34–37].
Hepatic intra-arterial chemotherapy	High concentrations of chemotherapeutic agents are delivered directly locally with the aid of implantable catheters [30,31]. Experiences with hepatic intra-arterial chemotherapy are based on regimens with fotemustine, cisplatin [32,33] or polychemotherapy [40].
Intra-arterial hepatic chemoembolization (transarterial chemoembolization)	This method is an extension of intra-arterial chemotherapy and it associates local high-dosage chemotherapy with tumor ischemia [30,31]. Cytostatic drugs (eg, cisplatin [30,31]) are administered directly into the metastasis through its feeding blood supply followed by embolization of the feeding vessel by occlusive agents (eg, polyvinyl sponge [31] or iodized oil [41]) that is placed via catheters. The retention period of the chemotoxic agent in the embolized tissue is prolonged by the blocked arterial blood supply resulting in necrosis of the metastasis [41].
Radioembolization/ selective internal radiotherapy	In selective internal radiotherapy and radioembolization, tiny microspheres of radioactive material are injected into the arteries that supply the tumor. Due to the small size of the microspheres, they are able to pass deep into the tumor vasculature, where they release doses of radiation to destroy the metastasis over approximately 14 days [30].

Table 5.2 Overview of localized therapeutic measures for liver metastases. CT, computer tomography; MRI, magnetic resonance imaging; TNF-α, tumor necrosis factor alpha. Adapted from 2013 German Melanoma Guideline [12], Kennedy et al [30], Agarwala et al [31], Becker et al [32], Peters et al [33], Alexander et al [34], Noter et al [35], Rizell et al [36], van Etten et al [37], Navarra et al [38], Bast et al [39], Melichar et al [40], Vogl et al [41].

Systemic treatment

The median overall survival for patients with stage IV metastatic melanoma is estimated at 8 months (± 2 months) with a wide interindividual variety [42]. Systemic treatment decisions should be based on interdisciplinary tumor board discussions. There is a general consensus that surgical therapy is the treatment of choice in patients with metastatic melanoma, if a complete surgical resection (R0) is considered possible. If it is not, and other treatment options discussed in this chapter are inappropriate, systemic therapy should be considered.

Chemotherapy

Adjuvant therapy after metastasectomy

No data exist for adjuvant therapy after successful R0 resection (no evidence of disease) in stage IV. Patient recruitment into a clinical trial should be considered, and alternatively frequent clinical and radiological follow-up checks are recommended.

> *Take-home message*
> A general recommendation for adjuvant therapy after metastasectomy cannot be made, as there are insufficient data to support this practice.

Monochemotherapy

Chemotherapeutic agents such as dacarbazine, temozolomide, carboplatin, cisplatin, paclitaxel, vindesine, and fotemustine have been tested as monotherapies in clinical studies in patients with stage IV melanoma (but without a placebo-controlled arm [12,43,44]). In summary, none of the therapies had a significant impact on survival time. The alkylating agent dacarbazine is the most extensively used drug in clinical trial settings and is therefore considered as a "reference drug" for patients with metastatic melanoma (Table 5.3) [12]. The latest Phase III trials described an objective response in 5–12% of patients. One-year survival rates reached approximately 35% [43,44]. Temozolomide is an oral alkylating agent that acts via the same active metabolite as dacarbazine and exhibits the similar favorable side-effect profile to that of dacarbazine. In Phase III trials, temozolomide and dacarbazine showed equivalent efficacy with regards to survival and response [43,44]. Common side effects of dacarbazine and temozolomide are generally mild and include fatigue, nausea, and vomiting as well as leukocytopenia, thrombocytopenia, and anemia [43–45].

> *Take-home message*
> Superiority of cytotoxic agent over another has not been proven yet. Monochemotherapy with dacarbazine is an established systemic therapy and may be offered to patients with unresectable metastatic melanoma if no mutation (eg, *BRAF*, *NRAS*, or *c-KIT*) is found.

Medication	Dosage	Frequency
Dacarbazine	800–1200 mg/m² IV or	Day 1 every 3 to 4 weeks
	250 mg/m² IV	Days 1–5 every 3 to 4 weeks
Temozolomide	150–200 mg/m² orally	Days 1–5 every 4 weeks
Fotemustine	100 mg/m² IV	Days 1, 8, and 15 followed by 5-week break; subsequent applications every 3 weeks

Table 5.3 Overview of monochemotherapies for metastatic melanoma. IV, intravenous. Adapted from Reproduced with permission from Leitlinienprogramm Onkologie (Deutsche Krebsgesellschaft, Deutsche Krebshilfe, AWMF): Diagnostik, Therapie und Nachsorge des Melanoms Karzinoms, Kurzversion 1.1, AWMF Registrierungsnummer: 032-024OL, leitlinienprogramm-onkologie.de/Leitlinien.7.0.html [12].

Polychemotherapy

A systematic review identified seven randomized studies that compared different polychemotherapy schemes with dacarbazine, with no overall survival benefit seen in any study. All combinations were able to demonstrate higher clinical response rates than dacarbazine monotherapy, but also significantly more toxicity [46]. Based on this, polychemotherapy cannot be recommended as a standard first-line therapy.

However, patients with a high tumor load, rapid tumor dynamics in either metastasis formation or growth, and/or progression after previous systemic treatment, present a particular therapeutic challenge that may warrant the use of polychemotherapy. In these cases, priority should be given to a temporary stabilization of the disease. Also, some of these patients enjoy a reduction in symptoms when treated with polychemotherapy.

At present, the carboplatin/paclitaxel regimen is most frequently used, as it demonstrated a progression-free survival rate of 4 months in a controlled randomized trial [47]. Apart from the stigma of hair loss while under therapy, patients commonly suffer from fatigue, and especially in the course of treatment, from sensible neuropathies. Due to the bone marrow toxicity, frequent surveillance of the patient's full blood count is required. Life-threatening hypersensitivity reactions may occur against the solvent cremophor [48].

> *Take-home message*
> Polychemotherapy regimens increase clinical response rates, but also cause significantly more toxicity compared with dacarbazine monotherapy. No overall survival benefit was shown with polychemotherapy.

Immunotherapy

As described in Chapter 1, T-cells play a critical role in antitumor immunity. Ipilimumab is a new therapy strategy that helps to augment activation and proliferation of T-cells, autoimmunity, and antitumor immunity. Activated cytotoxic T-lymphocyte antigen-4 (CTLA-4) is a negative regulator of T-cell action and thus of the immune response. Ipilimumab, a human IgG1 monoclonal antibody, blocks the CTLA-4 receptor located on cytotoxic T-cells [12]. Inhibitory binding of ipilimumab to the CTLA-4 receptor cancels the downregulatory effect induced by the CTLA-4 receptor (Figure 5.3) [49,50].

Two studies have demonstrated significant prolongation of overall survival in patients treated with ipilimumab versus treatment with a glycoprotein-100 peptide vaccine (10 vs 6.4 months) [51] or monochemotherapy with dacarbazine (11.2 vs 9.1 months) [52]. Severe side effects (grade 3 or 4) were frequently observed in patients treated with ipilimumab (up to 50%) [51,52]. As ipilimumab may induce severe immune-mediated side effects due to T-cell activation and proliferation, patients need to be educated that compliance with this treatment is required [49,51,52]. Side effects can involve all organs (the most common side effects are listed in Table 5.4) [53,54].

The US Food and Drug Administration (FDA) approved ipilimumab as first- and second-line therapy while the European Medicines Agency (EMA) approved ipilimumab as second-line therapy only.

As tumor response to ipilimumab may be delayed by weeks or even months after the commencement of treatment, tumor response assessment should only be evaluated after administration of 4 cycles (week 12). An additional whole-body staging is recommended to confirm a progressive disease, as pseudoprogression caused by influx of activated lymphocytes might obscure a potential clinical benefit of ipilimumab therapy.

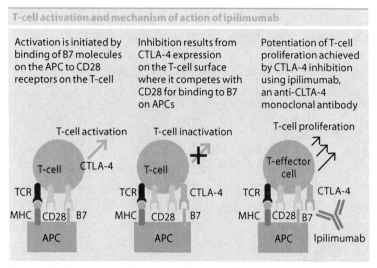

Figure 5.3 T-cell activation and mechanism of action of ipilimumab. APC, antigen-presenting cell; CTLA-4, cytotoxic T lymphocyte antigen-4; MHC, major histocompatibility complex; TCR, T-cell receptor. Reproduced with permission from Tarhini et al [50].

High-dose interleukin 2 (IL-2) therapy has been approved only in the USA and Denmark based on the results of Phase II trials that have shown enduring complete response in a minority of patients but no impact on overall survival [55]. Phase III confirmatory trials have not yet been conducted. IL-2 is hypothesized to stimulate antitumoral response of the immune system and is given in two cycles (Table 5.5). Response evaluation is usually performed 4 weeks after the second cycle. Courses of high-dose IL-2 may be repeated in patients with evidence of tumor regression [56].

Selected adverse reaction of ipilimumab

Common adverse events	Any grade (%)	Grade 3–5 (%)
Fatigue	31–41	3–7
Rash	8–29	0–2
Pruritus	11–31	<1
Diarrhea	20–37	1–5
Colitis	2–8	0–5

Table 5.4 Selected adverse reaction of ipilimumab. Other side effects include hepatic (hepatitis 1 to 2%), endocrine (hypophysitis 1–4%), and adrenal insufficiency (≤1%) and neurological problems (1 to 2%). Adapted from Yervoy package insert [54].

Major toxicities of this therapy include fever, chills, hypotension, increased capillary permeability, cardiac arrhythmias, oliguria, volume overload, delirium, and rash. Antibiotic prophylaxis is recommended to avoid bacterial sepsis. Due to the risk of multiorgan complications, administration is limited to younger patients with excellent performance status and organ function [56]. In the EU and the rest of world (ie, countries other than the USA and Denmark) this treatment regimen is not commonly used due to its high toxicity and the lack of data from Phase III trials.

Talimogene laherparepvec (T-VEC) is an oncolytic immunotherapy derived from the herpes simplex type-1 virus and is currently in Phase III trials for the treatment of unresected melanoma with regional or distant metastases. The OPTiM study, presented at the American Society of Clinical Oncology 2013 annual meeting, compared T-VEC with granulocyte-macrophage colony-stimulating factor (GM-CSF) in 436 patients with unresectable stage IIIB/C or IV disease. Treatment with T-VEC led to an improved durable response rate (16% vs 2% with GM-CSF), and an interim analysis found a greater trend toward overall survival with T-VEC (26% vs 6%). Serious adverse events occurred in 26% of those taking T-VEC and 13% of those taking GM-CSF; the most common adverse events with T-VEC included fatigue, chills, and pyrexia [58,59].

Take-home message

Immunotherapy with ipilimumab should be considered in patients with inoperable metastases (stage III and IV) and a life expectancy of >6 months. IL-2 is approved in the USA and Denmark but not in other countries due to its high toxicity and the lack of Phase III trials.

Overview of current immunotherapies for cutaneous melanoma		
Therapeutic schedule	**Dosage**	**Frequency**
Ipilimumab	3 mg/kg; IV over 90 min	Every 3 weeks (4 cycles)
High-dose IL-2	600,000–720,000 IU/kg IV (bolus)	Days 1–5 and 15–19 (cycle 1+2) every 8 hours; maximum: 28 doses per each two-cycle course

Table 5.5 Overview of current immunotherapies for cutaneous melanoma. IL-2, interleukin-2; IV, intravenous. Adapted from Bhatia et al [56].

Biochemotherapy

The combination of chemotherapy (either single-agent or combination) with interferon-α and/or IL-2 (so-called biochemotherapy) was not shown to significantly improve overall survival in patients with metastatic disease. Results of available studies with regard to benefit (response, time to progression, and survival) are inconsistent, as noted in the Canadian guideline [58]. Overall, the biochemotherapy regimens showed a considerably higher toxicity than chemotherapy alone, with the most frequent grade 3 and 4 toxicities being fever, chills, nausea, and vomiting [58,59].

> *Take-home message*
> Biochemotherapy is associated with high toxicity and is not recommended.

Targeted therapies

The commonly targeted signaling pathways and the targeted therapies are illustrated in Figure 5.4 [60].

BRAF inhibition

BRAF is a member of the RAF family of serine/threonine protein kinases. BRAF plays an important role as the main activator of MEK in the BRAF-MEK-ERK signaling cascade, a pathway responsible for normal cell differentiation and survival (Figure 5.4). BRAF mutations are detected in 40–60% of all melanomas [61]. Ninety percent of these mutations result in a single amino acid substitution (BRAF^{V600E}), while other BRAF-inhibitor-sensitive mutations, such as BRAF^{V600K}, are less frequent. The mutations lead to a constitutive activation of the BRAF-MEK-ERK signal transduction pathway, which is relevant for tumor development and progression (see Chapter 1).

The results of two randomized clinical Phase III studies investigating BRAF inhibitors versus dacarbazine in patients with metastatic melanoma have been published and have led to the development of the drugs vemurafenib and dabrafenib.

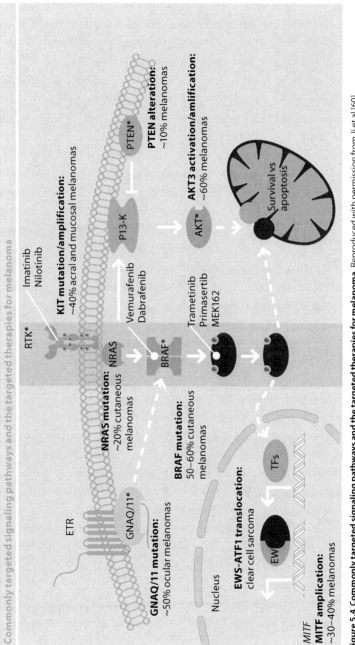

Figure 5.4 Commonly targeted signaling pathways and the targeted therapies for melanoma. Reproduced with permission from Ji et al [60]

In one clinical Phase III study, patients with previously untreated nonresectable stage IIIC and IV melanoma carrying a BRAF^{V600E} mutation were treated with the BRAF kinase inhibitor vemurafenib or dacarbazine [62]. The confirmed objective response with vemurafenib was 48% and progression-free survival was approximately 6 months. Furthermore, the treatment showed a significant improvement in median overall survival (13.2 months and 9.6 months for vemurafenib and dacarbazine, respectively).

A second pivotal Phase III study investigated the BRAF inhibitor dabrafenib versus dacarbazine in patients with previously untreated metastases and BRAF^{V600E} mutation, and similar results for the two drugs were demonstrated [63]. The confirmed objective response rate was 50% for dabrafenib and the median progression-free survival for dabrafenib, was comparable to that of vemurafenib.

The time of response to BRAF inhibitors is limited due to the formation of resistance mechanisms and amounts to approximately 5–7 months. The rate of progression-free survival at 12 months after BRAF inhibitor therapy is approximately 9% [64].

The recommended approved dose for vemurafenib is 960 mg twice daily. A dose reduction of more than 50% is not recommended. Dabrafenib was approved in the USA in May 2013 and is expected to be approved in the EU later in 2013; the recommended dose is 150 mg twice daily, approximately 12 hours apart, until disease progression or unacceptable toxicity occurs. In cases of low tumor burden or slow tumor growth/kinetics, ipilimumab (or chemotherapy) should be considered as first-line therapy even in patients with BRAF-mutant melanoma. BRAF inhibitors are contraindicated for patients with BRAF-wild-type melanomas (ie, melanomas without BRAF V600 mutation).

The most common side effects with BRAF inhibition (≥30%) include arthralgia, exanthema, alopecia, fatigue, photosensitivity, nausea, pruritus, papillomas, and squamous cell carcinoma (most commonly of the keratoacanthoma type) [65,66]. Prolongation of the QT interval is possible, and therefore electrocardiograms are required before and during treatment.

> *Take-home message*
>
> In patients with unresectable metastatic melanoma (stage III and IV) with BRAF-inhibitor–sensitive mutations, treatment with BRAF inhibitors should be strongly considered. Response and overall survival rates were shown to be significantly improved compared with the standard dacarbazine monochemotherapy.

c-KIT inhibition

c-KIT is a receptor tyrosine kinase for the stem cell factor. Activation of the c-KIT receptor leads to activation of downstream signaling involving multiple pathways, including the BRAF-MEK-ERK and PI3-kinase pathways (see Figure 5.4).

Clinical Phase II study results suggest that patients with a c-KIT-inhibitor–sensitive mutation may respond to treatment with a c-KIT kinase inhibitor, such as imatinib [67,68]. Progression-free survival with imatinib in patients with melanoma ranges around 4 months. The best responses to imatinib (400–800 mg/day) were seen in patients with a c-KIT mutation in exons 11 and 13. However, c-KIT mutations are seldom observed, most often occurring in acrolentiginous and mucosal melanomas [67]. The most common side effects of c-KIT kinase inhibitors are edema, fatigue, diarrhea, lack of appetite, nausea, neutropenia, and increased liver enzymes. In general, these side effects are usually mild to moderate. Other c-KIT inhibitors, such as nilotinib, are currently being tested in clinical trials.

> *Take-home message*
>
> In patients with a c-KIT-inhibitor–sensitive mutations, treatment with a c-KIT kinase inhibitor should be considered.

Medical management of brain metastases with targeted therapies

In principle, the same protocols are used for the treatment of brain metastases as for the other organ metastases (Figures 5.5 and 5.6). In the case of brain metastases, the blood–brain barrier is most probably not intact. Therefore, there is no certain advantage in applying anticancer drugs that penetrate the central nervous system.

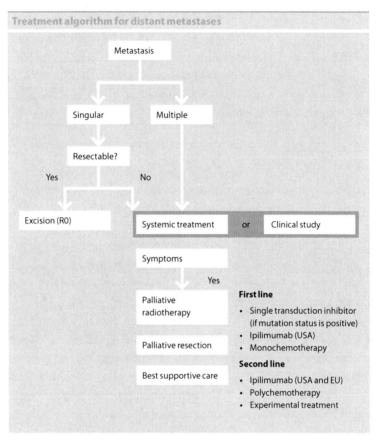

Figure 5.5 Treatment algorithm for distant metastases.

Clinical studies on the treatment of brain metastases are limited, as most studies in cutaneous melanoma exclude patients with cerebral involvement from clinical trials because of their low expected survival duration ($\approx$5 months) [69]. However, the available studies do not demonstrate significant difference in overall survival in patients with brain metastases treated with different chemotherapeutic agents. Response rates remain low (7–15%) despite systemic therapy, with a median survival time of 6 to 7 months [45,69,70]. The benefit of combination therapy also has not been demonstrated: sequentially administered dacarbazine and fotemustine produced low response in patients with brain metastases,

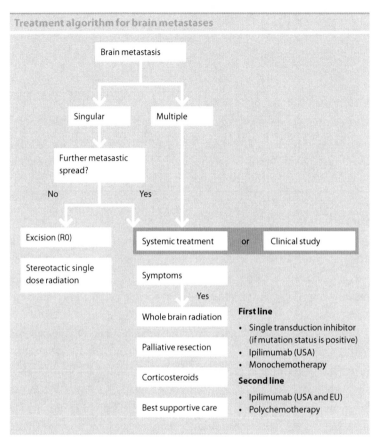

Figure 5.6 Treatment algorithm for brain metastases.

and the results were not superior to those obtained in other studies with fotemustine alone [70].

Due to the limited efficacy of cytotoxic therapies, new immunologic agents, such as ipilimumab, or targeted therapies, such as BRAF inhibitors, should be considered as treatment options, as the response rates observed with these agents tend to be higher. A recent prospective clinical Phase II study with the BRAF inhibitor dabrafenib included 172 patients with BRAF-mutant melanoma and brain metastases (study groups included treatment-naïve patients vs those with prior brain-directed treatment). A disease control rate of 80%, a median progression-free survival of approximately 4 months, and a median survival time of 8 months was reported for both groups [71]. Treatment with ipilimumab in patients with melanoma with asymptomatic brain metastases showed a central nervous system response rate of around 13% and a survival rate of 26% after 2 years [72].

> *Take-home message*
> Patients with brain metastases can be offered a systemic therapy similar to that recommended for metastases in other visceral organs. As efficacy of cytotoxic agents is low, preference is given to newer therapies (eg, ipilimumab, BRAF-inhibitors)

Quality of life

There are only a few reports in the literature describing a positive effect on quality of life associated with pharmacologic systemic antitumor therapy in patients with stage IV melanoma [73]. This can be partially explained by the long-standing lack of efficacy of the available medical treatments [74].

Impairment in quality of life was observed in patients with melanoma in the period following diagnosis and with tumor progression [75]. When metastases develop and patients reach an advanced tumor stage, they show an increase of the disease-associated symptoms [73] and, thus, a loss of quality of life [73,75]. Commonly-experienced symptoms include pain, physical limitations, nausea, vomiting, fatigue, and reduced ability to take part in social and professional life [73,75]. The aim of any tumor therapy should be to have a positive impact on the disease progression as well as on the patient's quality of life. This again emphasizes the necessity of an additional supportive therapy [73].

It is conceivable that therapeutics with an acceptable response rate and possibly a longer progression-free survival lead to improved quality of life, at least for a short period of time. Clinical data on quality of life of patients treated with targeted therapies are emerging and suggest some benefit.

References

1   Petersen RP, Hanish SI, Haney JC, et al. Improved survival with pulmonary metastasectomy: an analysis of 1720 patients with pulmonary metastatic melanoma. *J Thorac Cardiovasc Surg.* 2007;133:104-110.

2   Leo F, Cagini L, Rocmans P, et al. Lung metastases from melanoma: when is surgical treatment warranted? *Br J Cancer.* 2000;83:569-572.

3   Brand CU, Ellwanger U, Stroebel W, et al. Prolonged survival of 2 years or longer for patients with disseminated melanoma: an analysis of related prognostic factors. *Cancer.* 1997;79:2345-2353.

4   Manola J, Atkins M, Ibrahim J, Kirkwood J. Prognostic factors in metastatic melanoma: a pooled analysis of Eastern Cooperative Oncology Group trials. *J Clin Oncol.* 2000;18:3782-3793.

5   Morton DL, Mozzillo N, Thompson JF, et al. An international, randomized, phase III trial of bacillus Calmette-Guerin (BCG) plus allogeneic melanoma vaccine (MCV) or placebo after complete resection of melanoma metastatic to regional or distant sites. *J Clin Oncol.* 2007;25(18 suppl):474S. Abstract 8508.

6   Ollila DW, Essner R, Wanek LA, Morton DL. Surgical resection for melanoma metastatic to the gastrointestinal tract. *Arch Surg.* 1996;131:975-980.

7   Sanki A, Scolyer RA, Thompson JF. Surgery for melanoma metastases of the gastrointestinal tract: indications and results. *Eur J Surg Oncol.* 2009;35:313-319.

8   Pawlik TM, Zorzi D, Abdalla EK, et al. Hepatic resection for metastatic melanoma: distinct patterns of recurrence and prognosis for ocular versus cutaneous disease. *Ann Surg Oncol.* 2006;13:712-720.

9   Branum GD, Epstein RE, Leight GS, Seigler HF. The role of resection in the management of melanoma metastatic to the adrenal gland. *Surgery.* 1991;109:127-131.

10 Wornom IL 3rd, Smith JW, Soong SJ, McElvein R, Urist MM, Balch CM. Surgery as palliative treatment for distant metastases of melanoma. *Ann Surg.* 1986;204:181-185.

11 Mornex F, Thomas L, Mohr P, et al. A prospective randomized multicentre phase III trial of fotemustine plus whole brain irradiation versus fotemustine alone in cerebral metastases of malignant melanoma. *Melanoma Res.* 2003;13:97-103.

12 Malignes melanom: diagnostik, therapie und nachsorge. Arbeitsgemeinschaft der Wissenschaftlichen Medizinischen Fachgesellschaften (AWMF). www.awmf.org/leitlinien/detail/ll/032-024OL.html. Accessed June 20, 2013.

13 Eigentler TK, Figl A, Krex D et al; Dermatologic Cooperative Oncology Group and the National Interdisciplinary Working Group on Melanoma. Number of metastases, serum lactate dehydrogenase level, and type of treatment are prognostic factors in patients with brain metastases of malignant melanoma. *Cancer.* 2011;117:1697-1703.

14 Fife KM, Colman MH, Stevens GN, et al. Determinants of outcome in melanoma patients with cerebral metastases. *J Clin Oncol.* 2004;22:1293-1300.

15 Wroński M, Arbit E. Surgical treatment of brain metastases from melanoma: a retrospective study of 91 patients. *J Neurosurg.* 2000;93:9-18.

16 Overgaard J, Gonzalez Gonzalez D, Hulshof MCCH, et al. Hyperthermia as an adjuvant to radiation therapy of recurrent or metastatic malignant melanoma. A multicentre randomized trial by the European Society for Hyperthermic Oncology. 1996. *Int J Hypertherm.* 2009;25:323-334.

17 Seegenschmiedt MH, Keilholz L, Altendorf-Hofmann A, et al. Palliative radiotherapy for recurrent and metastatic malignant melanoma: prognostic factors for tumor response and long-term outcome: a 20-year experience. *Int J Radiation Oncol Biol Phys.* 1999;44:607-618.

18 Pyrhönen SO, Kajanti MJ. The use of large fractions in radiotherapy for malignant melanoma. *Radiother Oncol.* 1992;24:195-197.

19 Katz HR. The results of different fractionation schemes in the palliative irradiation of metastatic melanoma. *Int J Radiation Oncol Biol Phys.* 1981;7:907-911.

20 Herbert SH, Solin LJ, Rate WR, Hanks GE, Schultz DJ. The effect of palliative radiation therapy on epidural compression due to metastatic malignant melanoma. *Cancer.* 1991;67:2472-2476.

21 Dossgg LL, Memula N. The radioresponsiveness of melanoma. *Int J Radiation Oncol Biol Phys*. 1982;8:1131-1134.

22 Kirova YM, Chen J, Rabarijaona LI, Piedbois Y, Le Bourgeois J-P. Radiotherapy as palliative treatment for metastatic melanoma. *Melanoma Res*. 1999;9:611-613.

23 Rounsaville MC, Cantril ST, Fontanesi J, Vaeth JM, Green JP. Radiotherapy in the management of cutaneous melanoma: effect of time, dose, and fractionation. *Front Radiat Ther Oncol*. 1988;22:62-78.

24 Rate WR, Solin LJ, Turrisi AT. Palliative radiotherapy for metastatic malignant melanoma: brain metastases, bone metastases, and spinal cord compression. *Int J Radiation Oncol Biol Phys*. 1988;15:859-864.

25 Konefal JB, Emami B, Pilepich MV. Analysis of dose fractionation in the palliation of metastases from malignant melanoma. *Cancer*. 1988;61:243-246.

26 Sause WT, Cooper JS, Rush S, et al. Fraction size in external beam radiation therapy in the treatment of melanoma. *Int J Radiation Oncol Biol Phys*. 1991;20:429-432.

27 Suva LJ, Washam C, Nicholas RW, Griffin RJ. Bone metastasis: mechanisms and therapeutic opportunities. *Nat Rev Endocrinol*. 2011;7:208-218.

28 Bisphosphonat-assoziierte kiefernekrosen. Arbeitsgemeinschaft der Wissenschaftlichen Medizinischen Fachgesellschaften (AWMF). www.awmf.org/leitlinien/detail/ll/007-091.html. Accessed June 20, 2013.

29 Caralt M, Martí J, Cortés J, et al. Outcome of patients following hepatic resection for metastatic cutaneous and ocular melanoma. *J Hepatobiliary Pancreat Sci*. 2011;18:268-275.

30 Kennedy AS, Nutting C, Jakobs T, et al. A first report of radioembolization for hepatic metastases from ocular melanoma. *Cancer Invest*. 2009;27:682-690.

31 Agarwala SS, Panikkar R, Kirkwood JM. Phase I/II randomized trial of intrahepatic arterial infusion chemotherapy with cisplatin and chemoembolization with cisplatin and polyvinyl sponge in patients with ocular melanoma metastatic to the liver. *Melanoma Res*. 2004;14:217-222.

32 Becker JC, Terheyden P, Kämpgen E, et al. Treatment of disseminated ocular melanoma with sequential fotemustine, interferon α, and interleukin 2. *Br J Cancer*. 2002;87:840-845.

33 Peters S, Voelter V, Zografos L, et al. Intra-arterial hepatic fotemustine for the treatment of liver metastases from uveal melanoma: experience in 101 patients. *Ann Oncol*. 2006;17:578-583.

34 Alexander HR Jr, Libutti SK, Pingpank JF, et al. Hyperthermic isolated hepatic perfusion using melphalan for patients with ocular melanoma metastatic to liver. *Clin Cancer Res*. 2003;9:6343-6349.

35 Noter SL, Rothbarth J, Pijl MEJ, et al. Isolated hepatic perfusion with high-dose melphalan for the treatment of uveal melanoma metastases confined to the liver. *Melanoma Res*. 2004;14:67-72.

36 Rizell M, Mattson J, Cahlin C, Hafström L, Lindner P, Olausson M. Isolated hepatic perfusion for liver metastases of malignant melanoma. *Melanoma Res*. 2008;18:120-126.

37 van Etten B, de Wilt JH, Brunstein F, Eggermont AM, Verhoef C. Isolated hypoxic hepatic perfusion with melphalan in patients with irresectable ocular melanoma metastases. *Eur J Surg Oncol*. 2009;35:539-545.

38 Navarra G. Ayav A, Weber J-C, et al. Short- and long term results of intraoperative radiofrequency ablation of liver metastases. *Int J Colorectal Dis*. 2005;20:521-528.

39 Bast RC Jr, Kufe DW, Pollock RE, Weichselbaum RR, Holland JF, Frei E III, eds. *Holland-Frei Cancer Medicine*. 5th edn. Hamilton, Ontario, Canada: BC Decker; 2000.

40 Melichar B, Voboril Z, Lojík M, Krajina A. Liver metastases from uveal melanoma: clinical experience of hepatic arterial infusion of cisplatin, vinblastine and dacarbazine. *Hepatogastroenterology*. 2009;56:1157-1162.

41 Vogl T, Eichler K, Zangos S, et al. Preliminary experience with transarterial chemoembolization (TACE) in liver metastases of uveal malignant melanoma: local tumor control and survival. *J Cancer Res Clin Oncol*. 2007;133:177-184.

42 Balch CM, Gershenwald JE, Soong S-J, et al. Final version of 2009 AJCC melanoma staging and classification. *J Clin Oncol*. 2009;27:6199-6206.

43 Middleton MR, Grob JJ, Aaronson N, et al. Randomized phase III study of temozolomide versus dacarbazine in the treatment of patients with advanced metastatic malignant melanoma. *J Clin Oncol.* 2000;18:158-166.

44 Patel PM, Suciu S, Mortier L, et al; EORTC Melanoma Group. Extended schedule, escalated dose temozolomide versus dacarbazine in stage IV melanoma: final results of a randomised phase III study (EORTC 18032). *Eur J Cancer.* 2011;47:1476-1483.

45 Avril MF, Aamdal S, Grob JJ, et al. Fotemustine compared with dacarbazine in patients with disseminated malignant melanoma: a phase III study. *J Clin Oncol.* 2004;22:1118-1125.

46 Eigentler TK, Caroli UM, Radny P, Garbe C. Palliative therapy of disseminated malignant melanoma: a systematic review of 41 randomised clinical trials. *Lancet Oncol.* 2003;4:748-759.

47 Hauschild A, Agarwala SS, Trefzer U, et al. Results of a phase III, randomized, placebo-controlled study of sorafenib in combination with carboplatin and paclitaxel as second-line treatment in patients with unresectable stage III or stage IV melanoma. *J Clin Oncol.* 2009;27:2823-2830.

48 Szebeni J. Complement activation-related pseudoallergy caused by amphiphilic drug carriers: the role of lipoproteins. *Curr Drug Deliv.* 2005;2:443-449.

49 Tarhini AA, Iqbal F. CTLA-4 blockade: therapeutic potential in cancer treatments. *Onco Targets Ther.* 2010;3:15-25.

50 Tarhini A, Lo E, Minor DR. Releasing the brake on the immune system: ipilimumab in melanoma and other tumors. *Cancer Biother Radiopharm.* 2010;25:601-613.

51 Hodi FS, O'Day SJ, McDermott DF, et al. Improved survival with ipilimumab in patients with metastatic melanoma. *N Engl J Med.* 2010;363:711-723.

52 Robert C, Thomas L, Bondarenko I, et al. Ipilimumab plus dacarbazine for previously untreated metastatic melanoma. *N Engl J Med.* 2011;364:2517-2526.

53 Voskens CJ, Goldinger SM, Loquai C, et al. The price of tumor control: an analysis of rare side effects of anti-CTLA-4 therapy in metastatic melanoma from the ipilimumab network. *PLoS One.* 2013;8:e53745.

54 Yervoy [package insert]. Princeton, NJ: Bristol-Myers Squibb; 2012.

55 Atkins MB, Lotze MT, Dutcher JP, et al. High-dose recombinant interleukin 2 therapy for patients with metastatic melanoma: analysis of 270 patients treated between 1985 and 1993. *J Clin Oncol.* 1999;17:2105-2116.

56 Bhatia S, Tykodi SS, Thompson JA. Treatment of metastatic melanoma: an overview. *Oncology (Williston Park).* 2009;23:488-496.

57 Andtbacka RHI, Collichio FA, Amatruda T, et al. OPTiM: A randomized phase III trial of talimogene laherparepvec (T-VEC) versus subcutaneous (SC) granulocyte-macrophage colony-stimulating factor (GM-CSF) for the treatment (tx) of unresected stage IIIB/C and IV melanoma [ASCO abstract LBA9008]. *J Clin Oncol.* 2013;31(suppl).

58 Biochemotherapy for the treatment of metastatic malignant melanoma. Cancer Care Ontario. www.cancercare.on.ca/pdf/pebc8-3f.pdf. Accessed June 20, 2013.

59 Kaufmann R, Spieth K, Leiter U, et al. Temozolomide in combination with interferon-alfa versus temozolomide alone in patients with advanced metastatic melanoma: a randomized, phase III, multicenter study from the Dermatologic Cooperative Oncology Group. *J Clin Oncol.* 2005;23:9001-9007.

60 Ji Z, Flaherty KT, Tsao H. Targeting the RAS pathway in melanoma. *Trends Mol Med.* 2012;18:27-35.

61 Davies H, Bignell GR, Cox C, et al. Mutations of the BRAF gene in human cancer. *Nature.* 2002;417:949-954.

62 Chapman PB, Einhorn LH, Meyers ML, et al. Phase III multicenter randomized trial of the Dartmouth regimen versus dacarbazine in patients with metastatic melanoma. *J Clin Oncol.* 1999;17:2745-2751.

63 Hauschild A, Grob J-J, Demidov LV, et al. Dabrafenib in BRAF-mutated metastatic melanoma: a multicentre, open-label, phase 3 randomised controlled trial. *Lancet.* 2012;380:358-365.

64 Flaherty KT, Infante JR, Daud A, et al. Combined BRAF and MEK inhibition in melanoma with BRAF V600 mutations. *N Engl J Med.* 2012;367:1694-1703.

65 Chu EY, Wanat KA, Miller CJ, et al. Diverse cutaneous side effects associated with BRAF inhibitor therapy: a clinicopathologic study. *J Am Acad Dermatol*. 2012;67:1265-1272.

66 ZELBORAF [package insert]. South San Francisco, CA: Genentech USA, Inc; 2012.

67 Carvajal RD, Antonescu CR, Wolchok JD, et al. KIT as a therapeutic target in metastatic melanoma. *JAMA*. 2011;305:2327-2334.

68 Guo J, Si L, Kong Y, et al. Phase II, open-label, single-arm trial of imatinib mesylate in patients with metastatic melanoma harboring c-Kit mutation or amplification. *J Clin Oncol*. 2011;29:2904-2909.

69 Weber JS, Amin A, Minor D, Siegel J, Berman D, O'Day SJ. Safety and clinical activity of ipilimumab in melanoma patients with brain metastases: retrospective analysis of data from a phase 2 trial. *Melanoma Res*. 2011;21:530-534.

70 Chang J, Atkinson H, A'Hern R, Lorentzos A, Gore ME. A phase II study of the sequential administration of dacarbazine and fotemustine in the treatment of cerebral metastases from malignant melanoma. *Eur J Cancer*. 1994;30A:2093-2095.

71 Long GV, Trefzer U, Davies MA, et al. Dabrafenib in patients with Val600Glu or Val600Lys BRAF-mutant melanoma metastatic to the brain (BREAK-MB): a multicentre, open-label, phase 2 trial. *Lancet Oncol*. 2012;13:1087-1095.

72 Margolin K, Ernstoff MS, Hamid O, et al. Ipilimumab in patients with melanoma and brain metastases: an open-label, phase 2 trial. *Lancet Oncol*. 2012;13:459-465.

73 Cashin RP, Lui P, Machado M, Hemels ME, Corey-Lisle PK, Einarson TR. Advanced cutaneous malignant melanoma: a systematic review of economic and quality-of-life studies. *Value Health*. 2008;11:259-271.

74 Kiebert GM, Jonas DL, Middleton MR. Health-related quality of life in patients with advanced metastatic melanoma: results of a randomized phase III study comparing temozolomide with dacarbazine. *Cancer Invest*. 2003;21:821-829.

75 Cornish D, Holterhues C, van de Poll-Franse LV, Coebergh JW, Nijsten T. A systematic review of health-related quality of life in cutaneous melanoma. *Ann Oncol*. 2009;20(suppl 6):vi51-vi58.

Chapter 6

Emerging therapies and combination approaches

Apart from ipilimumab and the selective BRAF inhibitors vemurafenib and dabrafenib, which have shown prolonged overall survival and progression-free survival, several new targeted agents are being tested in clinical Phase II studies and are moving rapidly into pivotal registration studies. Only therapeutics that have entered a clinical Phase I–III study by the beginning of 2013 are discussed in this chapter. The commonly targeted signaling pathways and the targeted therapies are illustrated in Figure 5.4 (page 95).

MEK inhibitors

The rationale for using MEK inhibitors in melanoma is based on in vitro observations demonstrating an efficacy of MEK inhibitors in BRAF- and NRAS-mutant melanoma cell lines [1]. Several MEK inhibitors are currently in development, but trametinib is the most studied agent at this point. As the first MEK inhibitor in oncology, trametinib achieved a proof of concept in stage IV BRAF-mutant melanoma by demonstrating an improved progression-free survival (4.8 vs 1.5 months) and overall survival benefit (6-month survival rate: 81% vs 67%) in comparison to chemotherapy [2]. Rash, diarrhea, and peripheral edema were the most common toxic effects in the trametinib group and were managed with dose interruption and dose reduction. Administrative approval of trametinib has been achieved in May 2013 in the USA and is expected in early 2014 in the EU.

D. Schadendorf et al., *Handbook of Cutaneous Melanoma*,
DOI: 10.1007/978-1-908517-98-2_6, © Springer Healthcare 2013

In addition, the MEK inhibitors pimasertib and MEK162 are being tested in clinical Phase II studies in NRAS-mutant melanoma. Pimasertib is currently investigated in a Phase II, multicenter, randomized, controlled study versus dacarbazine (NCT01693068). Results are not expected before the beginning of 2015. MEK162 has shown activity in heavily pretreated BRAF-mutant (progression-free survival of 3.7 months) and NRAS-mutant melanoma (progression-free survival of 3.6. months) [3]. Recruitment for a Phase III registration study in the NRAS-mutant patient population is planned to start in the second quarter of 2013 (NCT01763164).

Combination of BRAF and MEK inhibitors

One of the first combinations that has reached clinical Phase III evaluation is that of selective BRAF and MEK inhibitors in BRAF-mutant melanoma. Recently published Phase II data strongly suggest that targeting the MAP-kinase pathway even more aggressively by combining both inhibitors can increase clinical efficacy with increased response rates with the additional benefit of reduced side effects such as cutaneous neoplasms. The most promising results of this study are that progression-free survival increased from a median of 5.8 months for dabrafenib alone to 9.4 months for the combined therapy with dabrafenib and trametinib and that the rate of patients without tumor progression at 1 year increased from 9% to 42% [4]. Administrative conditional approval of the combination of dabrafenib plus trametinib is expected for 2013 in the USA and in early 2014 in the EU.

Combination of vemurafenib and ipilimumab

In a clinical Phase I study (NCT01400451) conducted in the USA, the safety and tolerability of the combination of ipilimumab (an immunomodulator) and vemurafenib (a BRAF inhibitor) as determined by the number and grade of adverse and serious adverse events, is being investigated. Recruitment started in July 2011. Together with the population from a Phase II study assessing overall survival, a total of 50 patients with BRAF-mutant melanoma were targeted. However, no results have been officially reported, as toxicity issues have slowed down recruitment significantly.

This study was close prematurely because of unexpected, severe liver toxicities [5] and is therefore not recommended outside of clinical trials.

Independently, another Phase II safety study of vemurafenib followed by ipilimumab in the USA in patients with $BRAF^{V600}$-mutated advanced melanoma (NCT01673854) is currently aiming to recruit 45 patients. Recruitment started in the first quarter of 2013.

PD-1 and PD-L1 antibodies

The programmed cell death-1 (PD-1) pathway represents a major immune control switch, which may be engaged by tumor cells to overcome active T-cell immune surveillance. The ligands for PD-1 (PD-L1 and PD-L2) can be constitutively expressed or induced in various tumors.

Preclinical in vitro and in vivo experiments have shown that PD-1 and/or PD-L1 blockade using mAbs enhances tumor-cell specific T-cell activation, cytokine production, and immunologically mediated clearance of tumor cells. Two mAbs that inhibit PD-1 are currently being evaluated in various clinical Phase III trials in treatment-naïve and ipilimumab-refractory patients.

One mAb is lambrolizumab (MK-3475 or previously known as SCH 900475), a potent and highly selective humanized mAb of the IgG4-kappa isotype designed to directly block the interaction between PD-1 and its ligands. Clinical Phase I data suggest a response rate of around 40% in melanoma and renal cell carcinoma [6]. Recently updated clinical results have been reported on 135 metastatic melanoma patients, confirming these results and extended the clinical responsiveness also in ipilimumab pretreated patients [7].

Nivolumab (BMS-936558) is the additional mAb in advanced clinical development. It is a fully human, IgG4-kappa mAb that binds to PD-1. Based on results in 296 treated patients with various advanced tumors, the response rate was 28% among patients with melanoma (26 of 94 patients) [8].

Currently, it is expected that all clinical trials (NCT01721772; NCT01704287) will recruit patients globally into clinical phase III during 2013 and 2014, providing another excellent chance for patients to benefit from rapid drug development. The final study results and a potential drug approval are not expected before 2015.

Furthermore, first initial results of a clinical phase I study combining two immune checkpoint inhibitors—the CTLA-4-blocking antibody ipilimumab and the PD-1–blocking antibody nivolumab—appears to provide deep, rapid, and durable tumor responses in patients with advanced melanoma. Among 17 patients who received concurrent nivolumab and ipilimumab at the doses selected for further study, nine patients (53%) had an objective response to treatment, including three patients (18%) with complete responses. All nine responding patients had at least an 80% reduction in tumor burden at the time of their first radiographic assessment, by week 12. The overall response rate among all 52 patients in the concurrent therapy arms was 40%. As of February 2013, after a median follow-up of 13 months, 90% of responses were maintained. The estimated 1-year survival with the concurrent regimen was 82% [9]. A prospective randomized clinical phase III study, comparing ipilimumab versus nivolumab versus combination, is currently in preparation and is likely to start recruitment in middle 2013.

In a recently reported multicenter Phase I trial, the anti-PD-L1 antibody BMS-936559, a humanized IgG4 isotype antibody, was administered to a total of 207 patients including 55 patients with melanoma. An objective response (either complete or partial response) was observed in 9 of 52 (17.3%) patients [10]. A second investigational drug MPDL3280A, a human monoclonal antibody that also targets PD-L1, demonstrated efficacy in metastatic tumors, including melanoma, lung, renal, colorectal, and gastric cancers [11]. Of the 140 patients investigated for clinical efficacy, there was an overall response rate of 21%. Patients with melanoma had a 29% response rate, and responses seen were often durable, with 45% of patients still progression free at 24 weeks.

PD-L1 expression appears to be associated with clinical benefit, and further monotherapy and combination studies have been initiated. Although the immune system is capable of destroying metastatic cancers, it was not entirely understood how tumors evade attack. Recently, research has shown that tumors may utilize immune coinhibitory ligands, such as PD-L1, to dampen immune attack. By pharmacologically blocking PD-L1, tumor-specific T-cell immunity is restored.

Further clinical trials

The National Cancer Institute at the National Institutes of Health provides information about US and international clinical trials on its webpage. The list of current clinical trials and some general information are available from: www.cancer.gov/clinicaltrials or www.clinicaltrials.gov.

References

1   Solit DB, Garraway LA, Pratilas CA, et al. BRAF mutation predicts sensitivity to MEK inhibition. *Nature*. 2006;439:358-362.

2   Flaherty KT, Robert C, Hersey P, et al; METRIC Study Group. Improved survival with MEK inhibition in BRAF-mutated melanoma. *N Engl J Med*. 2012;367:107-114.

3   Ascierto PA, Schadendorf D, Berking C, et al. MEK162 for patients with advanced melanoma harbouring NRAS or Val600 BRAF mutations: a non-randomised, open-label phase 2 study. *Lancet Oncol*. 2013;14:249-256.

4   Flaherty KT, Infante JR, Daud A, et al. Combined BRAF and MEK inhibition in melanoma with BRAF V600 mutations. *N Engl J Med*. 2012;367:1694-703.

5   Ribas A, Hodi FS, Callahan M, Konto C, Wolchok J. Hepatotoxicity with combination of vemurafenib and ipilimumab. *N Engl J Med*. 2013;368:1365-1366.

6   Patnaik A, Kang SP, Tolcher AW, et al. Phase I study of MK-3475 (anti-PD-1 monoclonal antibody) in patients with advanced solid tumors [ASCO abstract 2512]. *J Clin Oncol*. 2012;30(suppl).

7   Hamid O, Robert C, Daud A, et al. Safety and tumor responses with lambrolizumab (anti-PD-1) in melanoma. *N Engl J Med*. 2013 Jun 2. [Epub ahead of print].

8   Topalian SL, Hodi FS, Brahmer JR, et al. Safety, activity, and immune correlates of anti-PD-1 antibody in cancer. *N Engl J Med*. 2012;366:2443-2454.

9   Wolchok JD, Kluger H, Callahan MK, et al. Nivolumab plus ipilimumab in advanced melanoma. *N Engl J Med*. 2013 Jun 2. [Epub ahead of print].

10 Brahmer JR, Tykodi SS, Chow LQ, et al. Safety and activity of anti-PD-L1 antibody in patients with advanced cancer. *N Engl J Med*. 2012;366:2455-2465.

11 Herbst RS, Gordon MS, Fine GD, et al. A study of MPDL3280A, an engineered PD-L1 antibody in patients with locally advanced or metastatic tumors [ASCO abstract 3000]. *J Clin Oncol*. 2013;31(suppl).